In this book Raquel Martin and Dr. Karen [...] basic ingredients necessary not only for good health in general, but specifically for achieving freedom from arthritis.

The authors' descriptions of nutrients, herbs (phytonutrients), exercise, body therapies, and stress management that can help are thorough and well-documented and referenced. In addition, Ms. Martin and Dr. Romano outline strategies for making the most of our present medical/pharmaceutical/insurance system and suggest ideas for compassionately making it better. But perhaps the most valuable contribution is the call for courage, personal responsibility, and discipline regarding our health care. Ms. Martin's personal experience attests to the fact that these qualities combined with knowledge can lead any of us back naturally to our birthright of vibrant health.

I enthusiastically recommend this book, not only for people with arthritis, but for anyone who wishes to explore new ways to achieve optimum health. I also recommend it to my colleagues who would like to learn more about nutrition and alternative or complementary medicine.

**Ralph C. Lee, M.D.**

As an educator in the holistic health field who teaches 200 to 300 new students each year, I try to keep abreast of the vast number of new books that are constantly barraging the health arena. . . . In addition, as both a naturopath and board certified clinical nutritionist in private practice, I like to suggest to my patients books that are informative, accurate, easy to read, and comprehensive in covering their topics. Ever since I first discovered Raquel Martin's and Judi Gerstung's book *The Estrogen Alternative*, it has been my first choice for books to educate both students and patients on the topic of alternatives to prescription hormone replacement therapy.

Well, she's done it again. In their new book on natural therapies for arthritis, *Preventing and Reversing Arthritis Naturally*, Raquel and co-author Dr. Karen Romano have managed to supply the reader with a very useable amount of information in just about every single subject area related to arthritis. This book is an astounding encyclopedia of information, and it succeeds in making unnecessary every other book I have read on arthritis. This one book has it all.

**David Getoff, N.D., Board Certified**
**Clinical Nutritionist and Educator**

# Preventing and Reversing
# Arthritis
# Naturally
## *The Untold Story*

Raquel Martin
with
Karen J. Romano, R.N., D.C.

Foreword by Joel Robbins, D.C., N.D., M.D.

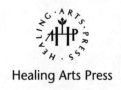

Healing Arts Press

Healing Arts Press
One Park Street
Rochester, Vermont 05767
www.InnerTraditions.com

Healing Arts Press is a division of Inner Traditions International

*Note to the reader: This book is intended as an informational guide. The remedies,
approaches, and techniques described herein are meant to supplement, and not to be
a substitute for, professional medical care or treatment. They should not be used to
treat a serious ailment without prior consultation with a qualified health care
professional.*
    *There can be great differences in the efficacy of various brands of products
discussed in these pages. If you use a brand at the recommended dosage for a few
months and are not satisfied with the results, you might consider switching to
another brand.*

**Library of Congress Cataloging-in-Publication Data**

Martin, Raquel.
    Preventing and reversing arthritis naturally : the untold story / Raquel
Martin ; with Karen J. Romano.
        p.  cm.
    Includes bibliographical references and index.
    ISBN 0-89281-891-3 (alk. paper)
    1. Arthritis—Alternative treatment. 2. Naturopathy. I. Romano, Karen J.
II. Title.

    RC933 .M346 2000
    616.7'2206—dc21

                                  00-039576

Printed and bound in the United States

10 9 8 7 6 5 4 3 2 1

Text design and layout by Priscilla H. Baker
This book was typeset in Janson with Stone Sans as a display face.

# Contents

# Foreword

Our bodies are remarkable creations. Treat them right, and they treat us right. Mistreat them, and disease is the consequence. The problem is that most people are unaware of how to properly treat their bodies so that they can operate as they were designed to—in health. And worse, we have come to accept that the aging and falling apart process is normal. Because most people mistreat their bodies in similar ways, most bodies fall apart in similar ways. Though this result is, in fact, *common*, it is not *normal*.

Further, traditional medicine is not helping in that it often only diagnoses a problem, explaining the cellular mechanism of the disease process and applying a treatment that addresses the problem but ignores the cause. Diseases and illnesses are not the result of drug deficiencies. I am all for using medications in life-threatening situations, but it is a crime to prescribe medication and subsequently think that all that could be done for a patient has been done. The worst thing, however, about drug therapy is that the patient does indeed get relief. Why is this the worst? Because the patient is sent home to continue engaging in the same lifestyle that caused the problem to begin with, only to develop another health problem down the road, for which another medication is prescribed.

We're missing the big picture of how the body was designed to operate. Diseases and symptoms are the body's effort to cope with being mistreated. Literally, the disease process is the body's survival mechanism in the face of some kind of mistreatment. Suppose you bought a brand new car forty years ago, and every time a part wore out, you returned to the factory to buy a brand new part to replace the old one. Forty years later you have replaced every part in the car, some parts several times. What kind of car do you have today? A brand new car that is forty years old. Now, suppose you were to replace each old part with a used part from the junkyard. True, the used parts are healthier than the worn ones you are replacing, but they are still used. After forty years of this maintenance approach, what kind of car do you have? One that is showing its age.

So it is with the body. If the proper nutrition is available to the cell—the car part in my above analogy—and there is no toxic interference, that cell can function in health as it was designed to function. It will repair itself as it needs to, to a state of full health, and when it comes time to replace itself, it will produce a healthy version of itself. But if the proper nutrients are not available to the cell and there is interference, then it will begin to slow down; it will not maintain itself in health and each new offspring it produces will be less healthy—your body will be running on worn-down used parts—ultimately resulting in a disease process. Drugs cannot reverse this process, only the body itself can—and many times I've seen it accomplish this.

As a doctor, it took me a while to figure out that I cannot heal a body. The only thing I can do is help my patients evaluate where they have gone astray in the treatment of their bodies and teach them a lifestyle that will give their bodies the opportunity to restore themselves. What this means is that each of us individually—rather than the doctor—is responsible for our own health. I tell my patients that we become sick for two reasons: ignorance and indifference. I can help with the ignorance, but each of us has to tackle the indifference by undertaking the lifestyle changes that are necessary to halt the mistreatment of our bodies, and instead give them what is needed for healing.

If we are to get healthy and remain healthy, we must take the initiative to educate ourselves. This is accomplished through asking questions

of health care practitioners, attending seminars and lectures, and studying informative books on health, such as the one you are now holding
in your hands.

It is with great pleasure that I introduce this work on arthritis to
you for it truly provides that which is necessary for any journey on the
road to health: education. Raquel Martin has done a masterful job of
giving the reader all the facts from a wide variety of sources, synthesiz-
ing these in a form that is easy to comprehend and apply. This book
does not pretend to have *the answer* to arthritis, for there is no single
answer. Rather, it provides a vast array of information from which readers can pick and choose to make their own decisions about what best
fits their particular situations. I know you will benefit greatly from the
information presented here.

Thank you, Raquel, for all your hard work and your obvious desire
to help others better themselves.

Joel R. Robbins, D.C., N.D., M.D.

# Acknowledgments

This book would not have been possible without the dedicated effort and the professional expertise of Karen Romano, R.N., D.C., my co-author and technical editor. Her broad educational background in a variety of health professions, her ardent desire to discover the truth about natural healing, and her ability to express in lay terms how and why we need to pursue preventive medicine were indispensable to this work.

For nineteen years Dr. Romano practiced as a registered nurse, which included intensive care unit and emergency room care, nursing home administration as both a director and assistant director of nursing, and home health care in Buffalo, New York, and Atlanta, Georgia. She has also served in the U.S. Army Reserves.

Today, she is a doctor of chiropractic who formerly taught nutrition at Life University in Marietta, Georgia. As we worked our way through the research papers and studies, her aptitude for interpreting complex medical abstracts in terms that could be understood by patients was invaluable. As an educator, Dr. Romano worked to provide an honest presentation of up-to-date nutritional information to our readers. On a personal note, her optimism and positive perspective during the unending rewrites and years of research sustained us to the end.

Anna Hyatt Perry employed her mastery of the English language to try to help us communicate an important message as clearly as possible. Toward that end, she initiated some major reorganization of this work. Her ability to absorb complex new subject matter was apparent as she mastered the rather tedious task of proofreading medical terminology. My heartfelt gratitude goes out to Anna for her patience, enthusiasm, energy, scholarly insights, and other multiple talents that she lent to this undertaking. It was a precious gift for me to work alongside someone who feels pure joy in just being of use in a meaningful task. This added quality brought a blessing to this work—a gift from above.

I am especially appreciative for the continued assistance and counsel provided by Judi Gerstung, D.C. Her background as a diplomate in radiology and doctor of chiropractic was integral to these manuscripts. She also contributed important research material in the areas of natural alternatives.

John Hart, M.D., was instrumental in helping me broaden my thinking about medical and natural health care options. His thoughtful, scholarly, and generous contributions were invaluable. He is a true ally in the fight for freedom of choice in health matters. This book is dedicated to doctors like him who have gone that extra mile to inform patients about preventive or functional medicine, which is so relevant in today's world of overmedication.

My deep-felt thanks also extend to Connie Smith for the time and energy involved in contributing information from her own resources on certain topics of this book.

My appreciation extends to Raymond F. Peat, Ph.D., who through his extensive research has brought us real answers to age-old questions about nutritional and hormonal balance. I have benefited much from his counsel via the Internet and am deeply grateful for his efforts in educating the layperson. My thanks resonate through several chapters of this book where I share some of his findings with the reader.

And space does not permit including everyone else who has assisted with this project. I am truly grateful for the many doctors, nutritionists, and other professionals who have helped me understand this vital subject and communicate the importance of addressing the causes, rather than the symptoms, of our disorders. They include David Getoff, N.D., Clinical Nutritionist; Ralph Lee, M.D., Ray Silverman, Ph.D.; Beverly P. Kapple, M.P.H., R.D.; John Hughes, Science Liaison and Reference Librarian, Pullen Library, Georgia State University; Jay G. Fromer; Sam Georgiou, R.Ph.; Irene Inglis; Roger Mason; Irene Steward; David Bundrick; Dr. Susan Starr; Mark H. Mandel, R.Ph.; Dr. Daniel O. Clark; Marcia Jones; Debbie Dombrowski; Susan LeFavour, L.M.S.W.; Dr. Cecil D. Laney; Dr. Daniel Clark; and most especially, Lee Juvan and Elaine Sanborn, my editors at Healing Arts Press. I'll be forever grateful to J. K. Humber, D.C., Wayne Neal, D.C., Judi Gerstung, D.C., and Linda Force, D.C., for providing moral support and keeping me in good health during stressful times.

And last, but certainly not least, there is the support I received from within my own family. To my daughter, Marie NyBlom, my love and appreciation for her generous gift of time and creative talent as she continues to maintain my Web page (http://home.earthlink.net/~marierm), helping me to reach out to many with the vital information contained in this book and others on today's health alternatives. Thank you, Marie, for your never-ending patience.

And my love goes out to my husband, Jack, for sharing his many gifts: the know-how and experience to find lost files on disks; execute contracts; perform last-minute revisions and edit the entire book to meet an emergency deadline; and upgrade my computer. I offer my gratitude for his sound judgment in the time of crisis and his endeavor to always aim toward tolerance.

I feel blessed to be working with Healing Arts Press, a publisher committed to health and well-being. My heart gives thanks to the Lord every day for leading me to all the talented souls listed above; for the curiosity, caring, and energy that leads us all to seek answers; and for the freedom of choice to put those answers to use.

# Introduction

Each year thousands of Americans of all ages who struggle with the effects of degenerative disease are told by their doctors, "You will just have to learn to live with it." Why, in this enlightened day and age, are we told so often, "There is no apparent cause for your discomfort," or, "It's just part of aging"?

Since the publication of my first book, *Today's Health Alternative*, and my most recent book, *The Estrogen Alternative: Natural Hormone Therapy with Botanical Progesterone*, I have come across more research showing the remarkable effect that natural alternatives have on "age-related" diseases and how they help destroy the toxins that end up in our joints and muscles. It was amazing to me to read the incredible number of *names* for diseases that are closely affiliated with, or possibly the same as, arthritis.

There is proof that a variety of botanical remedies exist that help to relieve, and even cure, arthritic conditions. Nothing conveys greater proof to me than the fact that these cures *work* for so many. When I find relief through natural alternatives, I write down the specific remedies so I'll remember to take them. How easy it is to forget in a busy and stressed lifestyle. Making lists has become part of my discipline— a reminder to put useful remedies to work. All my findings, however, developed into something even more significant than a reminder list. Sharing what I have learned about cures that have credible backing and explaining why and how they work turned into a tough assignment requiring a lot of discipline, but the end results were truly fulfilling.

While I was researching botanical progesterone as a natural

hormone replacement, clinical studies about natural aids in fighting arthritis also surfaced. What I learned made me realize that sometimes the penalty for ignoring nutritional hormonal deficiencies can lead to neurological and vascular disorders,[1] such as blood clots, strokes, and heart disease.[2] I also learned that specific nutritional deficiencies "sometimes are misdiagnosed as multiple sclerosis, peripheral neuropathy, and amyotrophic lateral sclerosis."[3] In the following chapters you will find a discussion of research documenting the fact that processed (refined) foods contribute to a variety of health problems including autoimmune diseases. Since author Paavo O. Airola, N.D. tells us that official medicine as well as the Arthritis Foundation assure us that "there is no cure for arthritis,"[4] it was gratifying to include this research for readers.

This claim has caused many to become dependent on doctors and drugs to relieve the pain brought on by arthritis and other degenerative diseases. The commonly used medications, nonsteroidal anti-inflammatory drugs (NSAIDs), disrupt and confuse our metabolism at the cellular level. Symptoms subside although destruction of the joints continue. When this happens, it is a real fight for nutrients (live foods) to adequately boost the body's immune system to allow the body to heal itself. Subsequently, debilitating conditions develop resulting in feelings of hopelessness and anxiety.

Also, once one begins to take prescription or over-the-counter drugs, it's easy to give up on finding the causative agent of the disease. In a state of ambivalence we don't readily attempt to change our lifestyle to one of natural alternatives. It takes commitment and effort; and in our weakened state we don't want to take on this responsibility. As I wrote in *Today's Health Alternative*, we may not have the energy, the willpower, or the courage to surrender our habits (routine lifestyle) to something new. We may have forgotten what it feels like to be really well.[5]

It's difficult to be silent after learning that there is a vast amount of essential health information available that's not attainable from mainstream medicine. This is why I'm speaking out—to provide freedom of choice, and a greater sense of confidence to those who seek alternatives but do not have the stamina to do their own research. In doing this, I have become increasingly excited about the incredible healing powers of the phytonutrients contained in plant-based foods. At the same time, I'm dismayed by the not-so-wonderful toxic drugs that are continually being prescribed—with no mention that the former have been proven worthwhile, or that they even exist.

There are many books that cover the subject of preventive medicine and do it eloquently and thoroughly. But the more I read about the notion that there is only one specific natural remedy that claims to be a "wonder cure" for arthritis or any other disease, the more I realized that it would be irresponsible to choose one therapy alone, and say it is the cure-all for everybody. Many natural therapies and non-toxic remedies exist, and, when used appropriately, they do not cause long-term, dangerous side effects, as their mainstream counterparts often do. The right regimen can take you on a personal journey to physical rehabilitation. This enlightened adventure can lead you to greater mental acuity and physical health, which in turn can provide the strength for spiritual regeneration.

I knew I had to share my experiences after learning firsthand how painful and debilitating arthritis is and then experiencing the amazing effects of a variety of natural remedies. I have tried to incorporate in this book a broad view of natural options gleaned from doctors, medical abstracts, and clinical studies. If you don't have the time or the means to attend health spas (throughout the world) so that you can be taken care of by the experts, this book can be a practical alternative.

In chapter 3, we discuss everything from the power of juicing and herbal remedies specifically for arthritis to the newest information on oils (essential fatty acids versus trans fatty acids) and the facts behind all the cholesterol misinformation. When I discovered what denatured foods can do to our body, it made me stop and wonder, "Do we live to eat, or do we eat well to live well?" If we wish to escape a life of pain, stress, and utter dependency, the latter choice is appropriate. In taking on this challenge, our goal is to prolong life in a peaceful frame of mind rather than prolong death in a painful state of mind and body.

In chapter 6 we will talk about some of today's holistic approaches that include natural hormone replacement for a variety of problems, including age-related disorders. We will discuss the true "mother hormone," pregnenolone, and its safe and natural use for arthritis. Emphasis is on rebalancing hormone levels rather than burdening an already stressed body. Conventional medicine offers therapies that temporarily suppress symptoms in the name of providing a cure.

You will find that the chapters on chiropractic (chapter 5) and medical alternatives (chapter 2) are vital to our main topic. Our goal is not just to live longer, but to maintain our health throughout life. Living longer is not a very attractive concept if the quality of life is not preserved or significantly improved.

So let's delve into the studies. We have no time to lose. Let's share with others so God, at the right time, will help those who help themselves.

# Part I

# Wise and Otherwise Choices

# 1

# Arthritis: Its Causes, Deficiencies, and Many Cures

*Physician, heal thyself—then you*
*will be able to heal the sick.*

**Paavo O. Airola**

There are more than fifty million Americans in the United States who are afflicted with some form of arthritis,[1] and despite billions of dollars being spent on the treatment of arthritis each year, the numbers continue to rise.

With today's hectic lifestyles, people have neither the inclination nor the time to study the literature that tells them how they could alleviate the health problems they live with daily. It takes a lot of effort to seek out and study research reports and, from that, to make intelligent choices. On the other hand, our current fast-paced lifestyles demand that we get help when we need it. When we're hungry and we have little time to cook, packaged foods and fast foods are readily available. We're on the fast track, a runaway freight train passing by the fields of fresh produce and missing out on plant foods that contain the phytonutrients essential to our health.

And when we're sick, a quick fix is always there in row upon row of over-the-counter medication or an easily obtained prescription. It's less work to follow the methods of traditional medicine, especially when they're neatly wrapped in an insurance package covering the bulk of the expense.

As we relax by the television after a stressful day's work, we are exposed to more than just entertainment. We see commercials that provide unending promises for "cures." They begin to take hold of our subconscious, stifling any initiative on our part to pursue better answers. We listen to the clever ads that say "wonder drug" or "new discovery," and we want to believe. These colorful messages tempt the mind with welcome solutions. Unfortunately, in our receptive state, we fail to realize the negative consequences these medications may have.

Nevertheless, when degenerative diseases such as arthritis strike, and our long-term use of these conventional drugs begins to take its toll, we ask questions. What type of arthritis do I have? Why are my symptoms similar to my neighbors, yet we were diagnosed with a different type of arthritis? (According to Ronald Lawrence, M.D., there are approximately one hundred names for the different symptoms of arthritis, or *itises*.)[2]

This book is not about treating the symptoms of specific forms of arthritis or discussing classifications of the disease. It is about prevention of underlying causes. Stuart Berger, M.D., emphasizes this issue by telling us how the symptoms of scurvy can mimic serious conditions such as bleeding disorders, deep vein thrombosis, and other systemic diseases.[3] This also applies to arthritis and all its invasive medical treatments, which could very well be lessened or avoided with natural preventive measures. We are still mesmerized into following the medical practice of dealing merely with the symptoms of arthritis, although studies continue to show that patients who are deficient in vitamins and minerals are prone to rheumatoid and osteoarthritis (as we discuss in chapter 3).[4]

## MASKING SYMPTOMS

The most common medical treatment for arthritis is nonsteroidal anti-inflammatory drugs (NSAIDs): Feldene, Aleve, Ansaid, Methotrexate, Indocin, Motrin (ibuprofen), Clinoril, Neprosyn, Fenoprofen, Vicodin, Meclomen, Celebrex (Cox-2), Advil, Tolectin, Nalfen, Oxaprozin, Voltaren, Orudis, Nabumetone, Elodolac, and many more will be added to this list in the future. Antimalarial drugs, corticosteroids, gold salts, and many other manufactured medications may also be prescribed. NSAIDs, as well as aspirin and acetaminophen (Tylenol), also have serious failure rates. For instance, Craig Weatherby and Leonid Gordin explain that "aspirin aggravates gout by raising uric acid levels."[5]

To initially relieve and temporarily mask arthritic pain, doctors write seventy million prescriptions yearly for these nonsteroidal anti-inflammatory drugs.[6] As many as two hundred thousand people are hospitalized each year secondary to NSAID use, while thousands of rheumatoid patients die from the use of NSAIDs.[7] Others suffer long-term adverse effects from other drugs.[8] John R. Lee, M.D., has the right philosophy when he says, "Your joint aching is not due to NSAID deficiency, and your doctor's prescription is merely treating symptoms, not causes."[9]

These drugs may temporarily reduce pain, but at what expense? As the body cannot assimilate these toxic substances they will eventually cause destruction of bone and joint cartilage. NSAIDs also cause severe ulcers, kidney and liver damage, and serious bleeding of the gastrointestinal tract. *The New England Journal of Medicine* informs us that long-term use of these over-the-counter drugs exacerbates asthma, allergic reactions, fragility of the bones, and immune system depression.[10]

Adverse effects from NSAID use are the fifth leading cause of death in the United States.[11] A documented study followed arthritic sufferers using NSAIDs and after twenty years over half of these patients became severely disabled or died.[12] There are, in fact, more deaths from prescription drugs every year than from "murders, auto accidents and airplane crashes combined."[13]

## SYNTHETIC HORMONES (MAN'S WAY, NOT NATURE'S WAY)

There are other prescribed medications that can eventually cause bone loss and arthritis or intensify an existing arthritic condition. Author Trien Susan Falmholtz states that "among drugs that increase bone loss and lead to a higher risk of osteoporosis are: thyroid replacement drugs; heparin (an anticoagulant); cortisone preparations (such as prednisone); aluminum-containing antacids; anticonvulsants; the antibiotic drug tetracycline,"[14] and some chemotherapy drugs.[15] According to *Prescription for Nutritional Healing*, James Balch, M.D., states that levothyroxin, a thyroid replacement medication, causes as much as 13 percent bone loss.[16]

## MEDICINE FOR PATIENT OR PROFIT?

In many cases, medications may be essential to treat acute or chronic disease, but prolonged use fails to correct the underlying cause. Although arthritic symptoms initially seem to go away when taking NSAIDs, the *disease* process itself continues. At first the medications deceive you into thinking everything is under control, because the symptoms improve. The side effects, though, hardly seem worth the price the body pays, especially since they sometimes become worse than the original problem. In addition, the underlying disease worsens over time, while its symptoms are masked.

The use of one medication often leads to the prescription of another to reduce the side effects caused by the first drug. These adverse effects are tolerated because patients are assured by their doctors that the appropriate "double-blind" studies were performed and the "seal of approval" has been given by the Food and Drug Administration (FDA).

Robert S. Mendelsohn, M.D., argues, "Most drugs are not developed to enrich your life, but to enrich those who make, prescribe and sell them."[17] And how many of us will heed the warning of William Boyd, M.D., who says, "If we continually interfere with nature, we must pay the penalty. Many . . . new diseases are iatrogenic [doctor induced] in nature."[18] An increasing number of people suffer from diseases caused by such medical intervention, and *iatrogenic* is becoming a more commonly used term among health care professionals and their patients.

Consider, for example, gold salts, one of many arthritic treatments. Gold salts can have side effects of blood cell problems leading to serious bleeding;[19] skin problems (ulcerations, hemorrhages); stomach disorders; deafness; anemia; neuritis; eye disorders; susceptibility to liver and kidney damage; and even death.[20] Paavo O. Airola, N.D., claims, "Gold therapy should have been abandoned long ago as a remedy for arthritis."[21]

## POLLUTANTS TRIGGER DISEASE

Serious diseases often stem from ingesting denatured foods—what is technically considered malnutrition. Nutritional foods and supplementation are not given much consideration by orthodox medicine. Simply "changing our diet" sounds too simple to be effective. In addition, sometimes it's more difficult than we think to put into practice what we know is good for us. Nutrition's essential role in preventing disease will be addressed in further detail in chapter 3.

My search helped me to better understand what I had initially suspected: "Arthritis is not a local disease of a particular joint but a systemic disorder, a disease which affects the whole body."[22] It can take years of physical and nutritional abuse to bring the body into this diseased state. Other major culprits that trigger disease are environmental pollutants (PCBs, dioxins, hydrocarbon, plasticizers, an arsenal of aerosols, truck and auto fumes); synthetic hormone replacement (estrogen and progestin); NSAIDs; chlorinated and fluoridated water; petrochemicals; personal-care products; and even plant and mold toxins. Exposure to all these exogenous substances can eventually cause allergy-like symptoms and altered immune function, which signal chronic inflammation.[23]

*reasons*

Poor lifestyle choices such as smoking and lack of exercise contribute to disease in the body. Bacterial, viral, or fungal conditions can produce complex ailments, which can in turn encourage infectious forms of arthritis resulting in trauma to cartilage or connective tissue. Jason Theodosakis and colleagues state that joints then become inflamed and "painful as the body releases enzymes that inadvertently degrade the cartilage as they seek to destroy the invaders."[24] Symptoms are a result of our body trying to eliminate these foreign invaders. So the cause of arthritis is not as mysterious as we're taught to believe.

*reasons*

Inflammation may be due to an external injury such as a sprained ankle, or it may be due to internal inflammation resulting from exposure to a variety of toxins. Julian Whitaker, M.D., explains that "edema may develop as blood vessels leak fluid into the surrounding tissues. Circulation is impaired, and pain and loss of function may follow. Immune cells rush to the area, and fibrin and other blood-clotting agents are formed."[25]

In recent years all of us have learned a great deal from adverse, and sometimes fatal, reactions to drugs.[26] More and more people are learning the truth and are seeking out safer and more natural alternatives to what has been traditionally offered. When you realize how the body can be assaulted by medications foreign to its cells, resulting in muscle spasms, nerve interference, and even nutritional or hormonal deficiencies—you are often moved to action.

Government is on the right track when they direct funds to cleaning up pollutants in the atmosphere and elsewhere. But there seems to be an inconsistency when we hear about the need to clean up the environment to protect our health, while the drugs we take may be even more toxic than the air we breathe. It's no wonder that the innate powers within our bodies don't have a fighting chance to heal us.

Addressing the cause rather than masking the symptoms is more logical, and certainly healthier. We are what we eat, drink, and breathe. "All diseases, regardless of their names, come within this understanding as only varied expressions of the one disease of **toxemia**,"[27] says author Stanley Burroughs.

Metabolic wastes are predominately stored in the connective tissue. This tissue is like the glue that holds the body together. When we regularly use antibiotics and other anti-inflammatory drugs, this storage area fills up with excess toxins. This can eventually interfere with the function of an already weak organ, joint, or immune system. Flushing out these toxic wastes with lots of pure water, fresh air, exercise, and good nutrition is a must.

Our future health is being formulated right now, even as we are being bombarded by environmental pollutants. With respect to some types of arthritis, Dr. Airola tells us in *There Is a Cure for Arthritis*, "Injuries and stress, per se, do not cause arthritis, but they may contribute to its development when the body's resistance is lowered."[28] Age-related diseases are the consequence of an accumulation of stored-up waste products throughout the body. Burroughs argues, "These toxins become crystallized and hardened, settling around the joints, in the muscles, and throughout the billions of cells all over the body."[29]

Those of us who have experienced the helplessness spawned by a disease and have felt it taking control of our body and life itself desperately seek out wiser solutions in the hope of reversing this condition. Suffering, fear, and frustration become catalysts that drive us to seek a better way to restoring health.

## RELUCTANCE TO CHANGE

Doctors are resisting alternative choices because they fear what they do not know; and patients fear doing anything other than what their medical doctor prescribes, even if the chemical drugs provide no more than temporary relief, and even when informed of the drugs' long-lasting side effects. Sadly, this reluctance to change can limit one's health, or even cost life itself. Trying to live longer through drugs is not a very attractive prospect. The quality of life must be significantly improved at the same time, or we will never enjoy the richness of human experience during our golden years.

With the judicious help of medical doctors, nutritionists, chiropractors, and educators, we are gradually enlightened about how we can avoid environmental and prescribed stressors. This is especially important as we age, because toxicity accumulates over the years.

## JOINT DISEASE (AKA ARTHRITIS)

*Arthritis* is an umbrella term for a variety of different names and conditions. Often, however, the root cause of the disease is the same despite the different labels. What is the common cause? *An immune deficiency.* This deficiency can be corrected through detoxification, and then healing the cells through nutritional foods, along with vitamin, mineral, and botanical hormone therapy if needed. A contributing cause of a weakened immune system can be nerve interference. The body often reacts to such disruptions with inflammatory symptoms. If we don't correct these causes, poor circulation will bring on chronic inflammation and, what is worse, the inability of the body to remove waste material or toxins.[30] At this stage of disease, the body must be cleansed of the toxic buildup. It is then that one can experience innate healing when pursuing nutritional and hormonal balance.

Although the cause of inflammation, or arthritis, may be the same in two individuals, their symptoms often vary, from muscle weakness, to connective tissue inflammation, to joint stiffness, and pain, and eventual immobility.[31] The following will give you an idea of some of the names of conditions that are joint and muscle diseases known as arthritis or are diseases with symptoms that manifest as arthritis. The conditions marked by asterisks are named by the Arthritis Foundation. Other names have been derived from references found in appendix B.

ankylosing spondylitis
Behçet's disease*
bursitis, tendinitis, and other soft tissue diseases*
carpal tunnel syndrome*
crystal deposition disease*
dermatomyositis
Ehlers-Danlos syndrome (EDS)*
fibromyalgia
gout
infectious arthritis
juvenile arthritis
lupus (systemic lupus erythematosus)*
myositis*
osteoarthritis*
osteogenesis imperfecta*
osteonecrosis*
Paget's disease*
polyarteritis nodosa*
polymyalgia rheumatica
polymyositis
pseudogout

pseudoxanthoma elasticum*
psoriatic arthritis
Raynaud's phenomenon*
Reflex Sympathetic Dystrophy Syndrome*
Reiter's syndrome
rheumatoid arthritis
sarcoidosis*
scleroderma
Sjögren's syndrome*
Wegner's disease*

Many of the sources listed in the endnotes contain elaborate descriptions of the symptoms of any of the above. One such book is *The Arthritis Cure* by Dr. Theodosakis et al. You may be amazed to find how many of the descriptions are similar to your own condition. As I read the symptoms of each one, I determined that I had a variety from several forms of arthritis—fibromyalgia, rheumatoid arthritis, bursitis, osteoarthritis, tendinitis, and one or two characteristics of some of the others. It's no wonder we come back from different doctors with a different diagnosis for the same problem.

## WINNING THROUGH PAIN AND LOSS

In searching for natural alternatives, I discovered that there are as many remedies for arthritis as there are types of arthritis. Unfortunately the natural cures are not usually available from conventional medicine. I therefore found it more productive to spend my own effort looking for holistic remedies and investigating why these worked, rather than finding out which kind of arthritis I had acquired. I discovered that when we focus on cleansing and building *host resistance*, rather than masking symptoms with medications, disease cannot exist. A healthy body doesn't get sick!

There is a need for a change, and it could very well be that we—as patients who have to live with illnesses and the side effects of medication—are the ones who will make this change. To survive, we need to become fit by raising our understanding above traditional medical dogma and going back to what is natural and pure for the body.

There seems to be no end to the unveiling of natural remedies for arthritis. Many of these have been found to be quite complementary to one another as they serve to promote joint and bone health. The more variety of healing sources that we can discover from nature, the greater are the *practical* results in health. In fact we are now hearing that *functional medicine*—finding the cause and dealing with it holistically is the way of the future.[32]

And because we are all unique individuals, we of course respond uniquely to different modalities. Some of us may have a positive response to one simple change. Others may need to explore a variety of techniques before healing can take place. Combining several remedies could even turn out to be a major step in determining an appropriate path to health. So, it might be useful to study natural alternatives before dealing with the pain!

## MULTIPLE THERAPIES FOR MULTIPLE SYMPTOMS

### An Alphabetical List of Choices

#### Bovine Cartilage

Bovine tracheal cartilage (BTC) has been found to fight inflammation and infections. BTC comes from a cow's windpipe. This cartilage therapy is effective and curative, with no incidence of toxicity, and without side effects.[33] It's a powerful anti-inflammatory agent useful in preventing many degenerative and infectious diseases. Studies have shown the dosage to vary anywhere from 750 mg to 9 g a day.[34]

The question often arises, Which one should we choose, shark or bovine cartilage? Here is an answer from *Dr. Robert Atkins' Health Revelations*: "I have never relied on a single substance to treat a sick person. My entire theory of medicine rests on the cumulative impact of a variety of natural substances."[35] His experience has shown that there is value in both kinds. This broad-based approach to the use of supplements may well provide an excellent guideline for us, too, when using natural products.

## Calcium

### Calcium AEP

This form of calcium protects our cells and improves nerve function. Dr. Atkins also found that rheumatoid arthritis, lupus, Crohn's disease, and early stages of multiple sclerosis respond to calcium AEP (CaAEP). Hans Nieper, M.D., a renowned German oncologist and cardiologist, found that this special kind of calcium "protects the integrity of cell membranes," and at the same time permits nutrients to enter the cell. Dr. Nieper has used it with great success on more than four thousand people. Dr. Atkins says that six hundred of his multiple sclerosis patients displayed "significant neurological improvements that run the gamut of the disease's symptoms, including less fatigue, less numbness, fewer spasms . . . better walking, strength . . . and improved coordination."[36]

### Calcium Malate/Citrate

When it comes to building bone mass, it's important to know which calcium we need to take. According to the *American Journal of Clinical Nutrition*, the absorption rate of calcium citrate/malate is better than calcium carbonate.[37] For this reason it is preferred by many nutritionists.[38] For reversing fibromyalgia, see the information on malic acid and magnesium later in this chapter.

### Microcrystalline Hydroxyapatite

If you're searching for a substance that aids in bone formation and absorption, look for hydroxyapatite. This compound appears as the active ingredient on more and more labels promoting bone health since it is the bones' most prevalent form of calcium.[39] It has been established that supplementing it is beneficial in decreasing bone loss.[40] Depending on the way it is processed, hydroxyapatite may actually have the ability to increase bone mass.[41] It should be freeze-dried (nonashed) bone from free-range cattle, and it should be free of chemicals. This form of calcium contains proteins, glycosaminoglycans, and a variety of other minerals and vitamins.[42] Researchers found that microcrystalline hydroxyapatite was effective in improving radial bone density, making it a valuable therapy in the prevention of osteoporosis in individuals with rheumatoid arthritis.[43]

## Cetyl Myristoleate

In 1970 chemist Harry Diehl accidentally discovered an isolated substance (cetyl myristoleate, or CMO) that kept mice from getting arthritis. When Diehl himself began to suffer the debilitating symptoms of osteoarthritis, he decided to use this naturally-occurring chemical on himself, and to his astonishment his swelling and pain decreased. After a few weeks he could hardly believe that he once suffered so from arthritis. Clinical trials (double-blind, placebo-controlled) with CMO have shown numerous benefits for those afflicted with various forms of rheumatic diseases.[44] Other studies were done with great success using two 75 mg capsules in the morning and evening. All patients showed improvement—even those who had crippling arthritis.[45]

Research demonstrates that CMO has an incredible effect on joint mobility. Anyone with arthritic pain who takes CMO will find an increase in joint motion since this nutrient possesses properties characteristic of essential fatty acids. In fact, CMO acts efficiently in relieving common forms of arthritis. It's effective because it "serves as a mediator of prostaglandin formation and metabolism; thus, CMO turns off the fires of chronic articular inflammation."[46] CMO is a major benefit in the treatment of arthritis and autoimmune diseases because of its ability to restore the natural lubricants within the joints.[47] CMO compound can be synthesized from beef bone marrow, fish oil, whale oil, and many other sources.

When CMO is used synergistically with some natural supplements, it becomes more effective in building cartilage and lubricating the joints. Such supporting nutrients are natural vitamin E, glucosamine sulfate, omega-3 fatty acids, and lipase (a pancreatic enzyme).[48] They all aid CMO in rebuilding cartilage that has slowly degenerated through the years. Researchers discovered that CMO was effective only for those who avoided alcohol, caffeine, and nicotine.[49]

## Chondroitin Sulfate

One function of chondroitin sulfate is to inhibit the enzymes that contribute to destruction of the joint cartilage.[50] Dr. Lawrence says that it "helps restore collagen and proteoglycans in injured joints." Chondroitin also stimulates an amino acid (hyaluronan). Dr. Lawrence continues to explain that it also "protects the building blocks of cartilage cells."[51] It has been found that chondroitin sulfate is nontoxic even in doses of 1.5 to 10 g per day.[52]

## Collagen II

We're hearing more and more about this type of collagen and its regenerative effects on cartilage and tendons. This protein is considered the "glue" that holds the connective tissue together as it naturally contains glucosamine sulfate and chondroitin sulfate, and "provides elasticity to the joints."[53] It also contains the highest concentration of mucopolysaccharides."[54] Harvard University School of Medicine found clinical proof that collagen II (even at the lowest dosage of 20 mcg a day) significantly reduced inflammation within the joints.[55] The most effective form of this nutrient is obtained from sternal cartilage of young chickens (six to eight weeks of age).

Other collagen II studies support its positive effects in fighting rheumatoid arthritis.[56] For instance, this substance was given to 274 patients who were suffering from this disease. After a 24-week double-blind study it was determined that it relieved joint discomfort and was a "potent regenerator of cartilage tissue."[57] This collagen protects cartilage from breaking down and at the same time encourages wound healing, inhibits joint degeneration, and even keeps the swelling down in damaged joints.[58]

Research has discovered that during the active stage of rheumatoid arthritis, "the body's immune system is attacking the collagen II in the joint." When we take collagen II orally, some of it is absorbed in the lymphoid tissue in the intestine. When white blood cells assimilate this collagen II, the immune system then suppresses the attack on our own collagen II within the joint.[59]

## Colostrum

Colostrum is the first fluid secreted from a mother's breasts after giving birth to a child. It is produced before the mother's milk comes in. Production continues for twenty-four to seventy-two hours and aids the baby's immune, digestive, and growth functions.

Baby calves also benefit from this whole food from their mothers. In fact, the essential components of minerals, vitamins, and antibodies in bovine colostrum are identical to those produced by humans. Colostrum is obtained during the first twenty-four hours of the second calving, when immunoglobulins are at the highest level.

The cow produces approximately nine gallons of colostrum. High-quality colostrum is obtained from cattle that eat green grass, not dried processed grain. It's essential that the animals be free of antibiotics, synthetic hormones, and pesticides.[60] This natural substance has gained popularity as a health supplement for a broad spectrum of conditions.

Biochemist Horton Tatarian, M.D., recommends colostrum for chronic inflammation and for a weakened immune system.[61] The growth factors available in colostrum can activate tissue repair of the myelin sheath, as well as connective tissue throughout the body.[62]

One study confirms colostrum's Factor-A stimulation of cartilage repair.[63] Other experts in the field of muscle fitness describe how the IGF-1 (an insulin-like growth factor) in colostrum is effective in building muscle. It slows protein breakdown and "stimulates glucose transport in muscle."[64] In other words, supplementing colostrum makes the muscles better able to utilize the fuel available to them.[65] Lance Wright, M.D., explains how colostrum can reduce pain and swelling and is even effective against many autoimmune diseases, including arthritis.[66]

Polish researchers discovered in 1983 that a protein chain in colostrum can indeed regulate the immune system. Futhermore, Daniel G. Clark, M.D., lecturer on quantum and molecular medicine and specialist in alternative treatments for chronic diseases, reports that immunoglobulins (a group of proteins that function as antibodies) from bovine colostrum have been effective in preventing bacterial and viral infections.[67] According to *The New England Journal of Medicine*, such proteins act as antibodies and have been successfully used in treating many diseases, including rheumatoid arthritis.[68]

## Copper

The *Physicians' Desk Reference* informs us that copper can be found in oysters, nuts, whole grains, and organ meats.[69] In her book, *What Your Doctor Won't Tell You*, Jane Heimlich tells of Australian chemist Dr. W. Ray Walker, who found copper chelates to have an anti-inflammatory effect, and that back in the 1940s and 1950s patients used this remedy to relieve their arthritic problems. "Dr. Walker also knew that the oldest medical text, the Egyptian Ebers papyrus recommends pulverized copper to treat various types of inflammation."[70] In some instances, "copper complexes are more effective and less toxic than drugs being used to treat arthritis," says John Sorenson. Some consider copper bracelets to be "a time-release source of copper that desensitizes the individual to irritants associated with chronic inflammation."[71]

Dr. Whitaker reports that "copper salicylate is more effective at pain relief than aspirin alone or copper alone." One study involving 1,140 patients given this type of copper showed "increased joint mobility, decreased swelling," and a list of other benefits as well.[72]

## Detoxifying

Detoxifying should probably be first on the list of cures; keep this in mind when you begin your pain relief and management program. Because of its importance, the various ways of detoxing the body are covered in chapter 3. Here we'll just touch on another method that will aid in removing toxins from the body.

Place one cup of baking soda (bicarbonate of soda) and one cup of epsom salts (magnesium sulfate) in your hot bath and soak for 15 to 30 minutes. This has a wonderful alkalizing effect on the whole body. Homeopathic studies tell us that it helps to get calcium back into circulation from joint deposits. I have personally experienced this natural and gentle way of eliminating pain. Enhance the effect by adding a few drops of essential lavender oil (or the essential oil of your choice). Often the simplest treatment can achieve wonders, and can do so much more efficiently and safely than taking drugs or undergoing surgery.

## Dimethyl Sulfoxide

Dimethyl sulfoxide (DMSO) reduces swelling because of its powerful anti-inflammatory properties. It is versatile and truly amazing—especially in treating arthritis. Studies have shown that this "exceptionally safe" substance "increases blood flow and oxygen availability to the injured area."[73] It has also been found to be an excellent remedy for spinal cord injuries because of its unique antioxidant activity (free radical scavenger), which aids in healing the neural cord tissue.[74] Rheumatologists, such as Salvador Charvarria, M.D., have found great success with it when dealing with the three major arthritides—osteoarthritis, gout, and rheumatoid arthritis. Other health problems respond well to DMSO, such as "sciatica, muscle spasms and spondylitis, tubercular and other vertebral inflammations, and lupus erythematosus."[75] Pat McGrady's book *The Persecuted Drug—The Story of DMSO* explains how this remarkable substance enters through the skin and is efficiently utilized in the bloodstream within seconds.[76] DMSO gel, rubbed into the skin, has even been used as an anti-inflammatory agent for professional athletes' injuries. Julian Whitaker, M.D., tells us it "seems to enhance the power" of other natural therapies. "DMSO is able to pass so easily through your skin because it bonds with water molecules both inside your cells and in the cell membranes." This permits the cells "to re-establish . . . normal and healthy balance." Some doctors find DMSO to be effective "as a vehicle for delivering pregnenelone," a substance that has been found beneficial in the treatment of spinal cord injuries as well as other neurological disorders. This will be discussed in chapter 6.[77] For my own use, I dissolve one of the many therapeutic herbs (capsaicin [cayenne], aloe vera, ginger, white willow, boswella, garlic, bromelain, or turmeric) into DMSO ointment and rub this directly on the painful area.

Dr. David Williams tells us that we don't hear much about this persecuted drug because it cannot be patented since it is made from a natural source. And even though it's been proven to work "in more than 3,000 independent studies that all firmly establish its power and safety,"[78] the FDA will not allow doctors to prescribe it.[79] For those who need more facts on its natural healing potential, information may be obtained by inquiring at health food stores, or through one's natural health care practitioner.

## Glucosamine Sulfate and Glucosamine Hydrochloride

Glucosamine sulfate (GLS) is one of the building blocks of cartilage as demonstrated in scientific studies. It can rebuild damaged cartilage and aid in reducing pain, tenderness, and swelling in joints, with no reported side effects.[80]

In a study of over one thousand individuals, more than 95 percent who were taking GLS showed positive effects.[81] Glucosamine is made up of glucose and an amino acid called glutamine, and has been found to provide integrity to bone and other supportive structures. Recent studies report that "glucosamine can halt . . . the destruction of cartilage by inhibiting reactivity to certain foreign agents, such as microbacteria, viruses, or allergens."[82]

Glucosamine does not cause gastrointestinal problems because it's absorbed so well in the body. Controlled clinical trials demonstrate that it is a beneficial safe treatment for osteoarthritis.[83] Other double-blind studies confirm the need for glucosamine sulfate.[84] Further research compares the efficacy of glucosamine sulfate with ibuprofen. After eight weeks, the results significantly favored glucosamine sulfate—especially in pain relief.[85]

According to Michael T. Murray, N.D., glucosamine sulfate has been the topic of over 300 research studies and more than 20 double-blind studies. It "has been used by millions of people throughout the world and is an approved drug for osteoarthritis in over 70 countries."[86] Further research shows that those suffering from arthritis are low in this important nutrient and that supplementation will be of benefit.[87]

Other studies say that cartilage-producing cells called chondrocytes are stimulated by glucosamine.[88] Dr. Theodosakis and colleagues state that pain is actually diminished by adding chondroitin sulfates, which aid in "protecting the old cartilage from premature breakdown and stimulating the synthesis of new cartilage"; so glucosamine and chondroitin together "enhance cartilage repair and improve joint function." According to them, glucosamine and chondroitin should be taken in two to four doses with food throughout the day.[89]

## Glutamine/Glutathione

This antioxidant aids and supports the immune system and muscles. Those suffering from chronic pain and inflammation have an excessive amount of cytokines (inflammatory molecules) in their blood cells. These free radicals are responsible for muscle wasting and joint destruction. Taking glutamine will encourage the production of glutathione, which in turn can halt the creation of cytokines that are so prevalent in people with rheumatoid arthritis and other autoimmune diseases.[90] Marc Rose, M.D., claims that "glutathione is one of the most important antioxidants made by the body, primarily in the liver."[91]

Your body can manufacture glutathione to fight osteoarthritis when you supplement with selenium (selenium dioxide, not sodium selenite). *The Arthritis Bible* reports that organic forms of selenium that are not normally found in food sources have "significant anti-inflammatory and analgesic benefits in arthritic patients."[92] Eating foods that are rich in sulfur (eggs, garlic, asparagus, and onions) will maintain the production of glutathione in the body. Glutamine augments the growth of muscle and obstructs muscle breakdown, and it may benefit people with lowered resistances such as those with autoimmune diseases who are on steroids.[93]

## Ipriflavone

This specific flavonoid helps to build and protect bone. It is known that isoflavones, in general, exhibit powerful antioxidant activity and can even "inhibit tumor cell growth by blocking activity of the enzyme tyrosine kinase."[94] Double-blind studies have demonstrated how this naturally occuring flavonoid can stop bone loss when used with calcium.[95] In some countries, such as Japan, Italy, and Hungary, one of these flavonoids, ipriflavone, is used for fighting osteoporosis. This natural compound actually reduces bone loss by its ability to "inhibit bone-degrading osteoclast activity." Japanese research reports that ipriflavones actually inhibit bone breakdown by "activating receptors on the surface of osteoclast cells." A two-year study showed that when participants took "200 mg of ipriflavone three times daily along with 1 g of calcium . . . spinal bone density increased 1.4 percent." Another study concluded that this natural compound not only reduces bone pain, but also increases immunity.[96]

## L-Arginine

This amino acid is becoming popular for its beneficial effect on bone growth with no known side effects.[97] It is now being "studied for its potential ability to slow bone deterioration and possibly encourage bone mass regrowth."[98]

## L-Lysine

If an arthritic person is having difficulty absorbing calcium into the bone, the amino acid L-lysine can help, because it promotes mineral absorption. A study done on dietary L-lysine and calcium metabolism in humans found that this amino acid should be used for prevention and treatment of osteoporosis.[99]

## Magnesium and Malic Acid

Clinical studies showed that magnesium and malic acid significantly helped patients suffering from fibromyalgia. The relief came within forty-eight hours of ingesting 1,200–2,400 mg of malic acid and 30–600 mg of magnesium.[100] Another study found that taking 200 mg of malic acid and 50 mg of magnesium a day was helpful for rheumatism.[101] (Other studies show the benefits of magnesium in cardiovascular disease.)[102]

I found a combination oral supplement called magnesium/malate. This combination has been found to be a potent aluminum detoxifier throughout the body and especially the brain.[103]

## MSM (Methyl-sulfonyl-methane)

This sulfur-rich mineral is found in cartilage; it will "maintain elasticity and flexibility."[104] Professor Ronald Lawrence, M.D., Ph.D., conducted a double-blind study and reported that patients suffering from degenerative arthritis who took MSM on a daily basis experienced as much as 80 percent pain relief.[105] It has been found that taking this organic sulfur as a supplement can also alleviate the discomforts of many other illnesses.[106] In addition, MSM is safe, as it is obtained from a variety of raw foods.

Although a member of the sul*fur* family, it should not be grouped with sul*fa* drugs, to which some people are allergic,[107] or to sul*fites*, which are used in many processed foods as additives. Sulfites can be dangerous to our health—destroying important vitamins, causing asthmatic conditions, and exacerbating allergies. Sul*fur* is essential for the muscles, skin, and bones. It aids in the manufacture of collagen and is "the primary constituent of cartilage and connective tissue."[108] A deficiency in sulfur would affect every cell in the body and cause pain and even disease.

Do you know people who predict weather changes based on their joint pain? Dr. Earl L. Mindell explains why some people's bodies react to changes of temperature in his book *The MSM Miracle*: "Often, what contributes to the pain is the lack of flexibility and permeability in the fibrous tissue cells. Use of MSM has been shown to add flexibility to cell walls while allowing fluids to pass through the tissue more easily. This softens the tissue and helps to equalize pressure thereby reducing if not totally eliminating the cause of the pain."[109]

As MSM allows harmful toxins such as lactic acid to flow out of the cells, it permits nutrients to flow in.[110] Due to its variety of benefits in the body, it actually improves overall health.[111] Long-lasting relief has been found with dosages anywhere from 100 mg to as much as 5,000 mg.[112] For optimum relief from the pain associated with osteoarthritis, bursitis, and other types of joint pain, it has been suggested that a supplement consisting of glucosamine with MSM might be effective.[113] Consistent use of MSM has been found to relieve pain as well as Motrin, but without side effects.[114]

## OPCs (Grape Seed Extract/Pine Bark)

Many doctors are using this active bioflavonoid from grapeseed and maritime pine bark extract to fight infections and combat inflammation. It is considered to be "fifty times stronger than vitamin E, [and] 20 times stronger than vitamin C."[115] Early research proved this to be effective for capillary fragility and joint disorders. As an antioxidant it can help to neutralize free radicals by protecting collagen from excess collagenase (an enzyme that destroys collagen). It also assists vitamin C in making new and healthier collagen.[116] Because of its anti-inflammatory action, *The Arthritis Bible* suggests that it "should be considered as a promising therapeutic agent for osteoarthritis and inflammatory rheumatic diseases.[117]

The above combination aids in resisting inflammation and improves circulation and joint flexibility.[118] Dr. Robert D. Willix Jr. also confirms that this extract possesses "properties that stabilize and maintain the integrity of blood vessels and provide collagen support. Dr. Willix recommends it for inflammation associated with arthritis and sports injuries.[119]

## SAMe (S-adenosyl-methionine)

This compound is mostly manufactured in the liver where it is used to detoxify the body of pollutants such as drugs, pesticides, alcohol, and solvents.[120] Our body manufactures SAMe from an amino acid (methionine) obtained from protein foods. Difficulties with protein digestion would obviously lead to deficiencies in this important substance. Substituting with B vitamins, particularly $B_{12}$ and folic acid,[121] will help to maintain the methionine.[122] This molecule regulates gene performance, aids in the insulating of cells, and manages hormones and neurotransmitters (serotonin, adrenaline, melatonin, and dopamine). SAMe is sometimes referred to as a "methyl donor" and is found in every living cell in our body.

SAMe is reported to preserve and even restore cartilage.[123] Author

Sol Grazi, M.D., further explains that it not only encourages cartilage growth, but it also is without any of the side effects that have been attributed to other arthritis medications such as the NSAIDs, which "contribute to cartilage deterioration." SAMe's greatest use to the body is in its "ability to transfer sulfur, which is used to make cysteine, taurine, and glutathione, all important substances for metabolism."[124] *The Arthritis Bible* explains that "SAMe increases cellular production and blood levels of proteoglycans—the building blocks of cartilage."[125]

This biological compound was actually discovered in Italy in 1952. Trials in England and Sweden found supplementing with SAMe provided relief from pain and stiffness relating to conditions of arthritis.[126] Dr. Grazi tells us that SAMe helps in osteoarthritis more than any other form of arthritis. It significantly decreases pain in the joints such as the knees, hips, jaw, neck, and fingers—where there tends to be swelling, stiffness, or deformity.[127] *The British Journal of Rheumatology*[128] and *The American Journal of Medicine* found similar therapeutic effects in treating osteoarthritis in their study involving twenty-two thousand patients. A variety of studies explain its influence on fibromyalgia.[129] Dr. Grazi describes its therapeutic value in treating liver disease and how it repairs and reverses injury done to the liver. He also tells us that it has been used to treat a variety of forms of depression.[130]

This natural over-the-counter amino acid supplement is best absorbed through the intestines. Optimal results are achieved when you take these tablets in an enteric, coated form and on an empty stomach.[131] SAMe therapy has brought relief to thousands of patients in the fight against many physical and mental diseases.[132]

## Shark Cartilage

Cartilage extracts stimulate protein and chondroitin-sulfate synthesis.[133] So, if you eat cartilage, this will promote stronger cartilage—according to the homeopathic principle that "like cures like."[134]

Mucopolysaccharides, the complex carbohydrates in shark carti-lage, benefit the immune system and reduce the inflammation and pain associated with arthritis.[135] Dr. I. William Lane, in his book *Sharks Don't Get Cancer*, reports that shark cartilage is not only "effective against arthritis," but is a "therapy that can be used to treat a host of dis-eases."[136] Dr. Atkins used about 70 g of shark cartilage a day and saw how this supplement contributed to healing not only rheumatism and osteoarthritis, but also allergies, infections, and even the Epstein-Barr virus.[137] It's also known to "shut off blood vessel growth to abnormal tumors and generate new blood vessels in scar tissue."[138]

### Silica

Some rheumatologists prescribe silica gel to restore tissue elasticity. This gel prevents bone decalcification and is helpful for "the preven-tion of osteoporosis, especially for women beyond the age of 35 years."[139] Silica can be found in an organic form as a colloidal mineral. It has been found beneficial in supporting the immune system.[140]

A friend of mine had a painful bone spur on her heel. She was in-structed to take a silica tablet before bedtime for ten days. This and other homeopathic remedies are more effective if no food is ingested before or after they're administered. At first the pain seemed to get worse, but every day she became less aware of the discomfort, and by the ninth day the pain and swelling were gone.

### *Miscellaneous Arthritis Remedies*

Other important supplements that have anti-inflammatory effects are chlorophyll, thymus gland extract, capsaicin, and pantothenic acid.[141]

Quercetin, a bioflavonoid, subdues the production of two inflam-matory agents: leukotrienes and histamines. Taking bromelain with quercetin results in the best "synergistic anti-inflammatory activity."[142] Coenzyme Q10, a powerful anti-oxidant, can be supplemented (as the body's production of it declines with age) to improve circulation and provide energy. It acts much as vitamin E does.[143] Stephen T. Sinatra, M.D., explains that "Coenzyme Q10 works to stabilize the membrane, thus preventing cellular breakdown in your joints."[144] Zinc sulfate is effective in treating rheumatoid arthritis because of its mild anti-inflammatory property.[145] It should always be supplemented with copper for proper absorption. Other studies explain zinc's effectiveness in combating inflammation and stiffness in rheumatoid arthritis.[146] Ginseng boosts the immune system by aiding balance and adrenal support. More information on herbs and enzymes that have been found to have a direct role in combating arthritic conditions is given in chapters 2 and 3.

## Chelation

When preventive care has not been a part of a person's way of life, degenerative diseases often get out of hand and more extreme treatment may be warranted. Dr. Morton Walker explains that when conditions such as arthritis or cases of calcium deposits become severe, intravenous chelation therapy is most effective for removing deposits of calcium. It must be administered under a chelation physician's supervision.[147] Oral chelation foods are whole-grain wheat, bran, oats, corn, cereals, lentils, beans, peas, fresh fruit and vegetables, nuts, seeds, and other rich sources of fiber.[148] For more information on chelation, see studies listed in appendix B.

## Exercise

One of the most beneficial activities we can provide ourselves is simple daily walks. We will not only strengthen the cardiovascular system, but also capture vitamin D, the "sunshine vitamin." Vitamin D aids calcium in building bone density.[149] Because of this, a vitamin D deficiency can cause many health problems, including arthritis symptoms, slow healing, muscle cramps,[150] and osteoporosis.

Physical activity is vital to healthy living. It improves muscle strength, builds stamina, and allows joints to move more easily, with less pain and swelling. Regardless of the type or severity of arthritis, there are appropriate forms of exercise that can provide benefits without harming the joints.

In rheumatoid arthritis, the lining of the synovial capsule within the joint becomes inflamed. The inflammation causes breakdown and swelling of the synovial tissue and weakens the tendons, ligaments, and joint capsule. Synovial fluid decreases in quality, inhibiting nourishing cleansing and lubrication of the joint while the lining of the capsule overgrows in an attempt to heal. The joint weakens and ultimately stiffens, unless the process is reversed. In osteoarthritis, degenerative processes begin in the joint or disc space and can spread to the nearby bone. These changes often lead to the formation of bone spurs (excess bone) that painfully grate on other bone.

Exercise induces the manufacture of synovial fluid and circulates it throughout the entire joint space. This increases circulation of both the blood and lymphatic systems, which ultimately reduces swelling, removes waste products, and increases the delivery of oxygen and nutrients for joint healing. Exercise also strengthens shock-absorbing muscles and ligaments around the joints, taking pressure off the joints.

The key to an arthritis exercise program is to increase joint flexibility, muscle strength, and stamina, without putting undue stress on the joints. Recommendations include range-of-motion exercises, strengthening exercises, stretching, and aerobics. Your choice of exercise is a personal one. It may include bicycling, walking, martial arts, swimming, cross-country skiing, rowing, or water exercises. Yoga has been found to be helpful as it strengthens the muscles and joints through stretching. Even if some joints are too painful to exercise during arthritis flare-ups, gentle stretching maintains healthy muscles, tendons, ligaments, and bones, and improves mobility of the joints themselves.

Physical overexertion has been known to shorten life expectancy by producing free radicals and premature degeneration at the cellular level. Because of this, Chinese martial arts such as tai chi or chi kung offer an advantage over many Western-style sports. Chi kung has a calming effect on the whole nervous system and at the same time "stimulates the immune system and is favorable for the healing of inflamed or degenerated tissue," according to Yves Requen, author of *Chi Kung: The Chinese Art of Mastering Energy*.[151] This could be because these exercises strengthen one's physical and mental powers by opening the energy pathways (meridians) throughout the body. As the body continues to move in stretching and flexing movements, circulation is enhanced, strengthening the spirit and life within the body, and "disease cannot find a place to settle." Chi kung is a perfect exercise for those suffering from arthritic conditions because it stimulates the twelve meridians and firms muscle tone. For instance, one of the powerful yet stress-free exercises in chi kung is called *embracing the tree*. It opens all the meridians so that energy circulates freely throughout all the body systems, including the muscles, skin, bones, organs, and brain. This exercise aids in toxin elimination and increases immunity needed for fighting many diseases, including osteoarthritis.

Older people with physical disabilities are helped through chi kung as joints and muscles become less stiff and finally pain free. Chi kung is a potent and effective way of aiding those suffering from rheumatism.

A final thought on this subject: Be sure to pick an exercise that makes you feel alive and happy. If you're the type who gets flustered because you can't keep up with the group in your classes, obtain a dance video specifically for arthritis sufferers so you can exercise at your own pace and in the privacy of your own home. If you feel more disciplined with a group, invite friends and other kindred spirits who share your same needs. Dance methods can be modified to lower impact, and they can help your flexibility and posture. Dance can provide range-of-motion, endurance, and repetition training; and it can lift the spirit and drive away depression.[152] Choosing your own background music will certainly help prevent the boredom that sometimes sets in with a workout routine. With all this, keep in mind that "staying in shape . . . [is] not only a personal quest, but a spiritual imperative."[153]

## Water (Purified/Distilled)

Dehydration can contribute to arthritis. Joint cartilage suffers when there is a shortage of water. F. Batmanghelidj, M.D., argues, "Rheumatoid joint pain is a direct signal of . . . water deficiency." Water is essential to life, and, in its pure form, to health. Dr. Batmanghelidj explains why arthritis and other diseases are often caused by chronic dehydration. One of the first things to try when you encounter the pain of arthritis, backaches, headaches, and stomach and intestinal disorders is to nourish the body with generous amounts of water. You may be amazed at the results. Dr. Batmanghelidj warns us *not to treat thirst with medication*, explaining that pure water will bring about cell-volume balance in the body and result in more efficient cell activity.[154]

When the body is in a dehydrated state, enzymes and proteins are not as efficient. Dr. Batmanghelidj says, "The damage occurs at a level of persistent dehydration that does not necessarily demonstrate a 'dry mouth signal.'" So it's important that we drink pure water throughout the day. If we wait till we're thirsty, our cells have already suffered. The swelling of joints will often disappear when the joint becomes hydrated, and the joint structure itself will begin to mend.[155]

Many health professionals recommend we drink approximately one-half ounce of water a day for every pound of body weight. Make sure, however, that it's distilled water fortified with liquid minerals. Health pioneer Paul Bragg tells us that drinking distilled water flushes out mineral deposits from various parts of the body and cholesterol from our arteries.[156] Tap water contains these inorganic minerals as well as

*Tap water risks.*

approximately seven hundred other chemicals (129 of which are cited by the Environmental Protection Agency as causing serious health risks).[157] In his book *Water Can Undermine Your Health*, Dr. Norman W. Walker explains that if water is not distilled, inorganic calcium (lime), magnesium, and other inorganic minerals cannot be utilized by the body.[158] Dr. George H. Malkmus says that what is not eliminated can accumulate in the body and cause stiffness in the joints.[159]

Distillation (or reverse osmosis) is as close as we can get to nature's form of water purification. Also, the 212-degree heat in a stainless steel condenser produces steam that is free from impurities and chemicals; the heat also kills bacteria and viruses. Alternative water treatments using filters can be breeding grounds for bacteria. Filtering attempts to "remove contaminants from water, rather than removing water from the contaminants."[160]

Dr. Batmanghelidj, author of a variety of research papers on water metabolism and pain, shows how cells throughout the body, and within the bone, depend most particularly on water.[161] He tells us that chronic pain is a sign of chronic dehydration and "rheumatoid joint pain is a direct signal of local water deficiency of the body."[162] In his book on how to deal with arthritis, he discusses how this can lead to damaged cartilage.[163] Patients who have found relief through his diet and stretching program applaud his research, which recognizes the regulatory and reactive hydrolytic functions of water in the body.[164]

As we get older, we need more water, yet the thirst sensation is decreased, and thus level of thirst is not a reliable indicator of chronic dehydration.[165] We normally consume water quickly and without thought to whether our bodies have had enough. But when we drink more than our thirst calls for, proteins are used more efficiently.[166] Putting Dr. Batmanghelidj's investigation into practice seems to be a sensible way to fight disease and avoid pain.

## ONE REMEDY ALONE IS NOT A PERMANENT SOLUTION

Any of the above options used *alone* without incorporating a proper overall nutritional program will not bring optimum health. This is especially true when we consider the added burden of dealing with the daily stresses of life. Doctors who specialize in natural healing realize that dietary modifications and lifestyle changes are an essential part of the solution.

With so many natural remedies and treatments available today, we can choose the ones that work for us. Every body has distinctive needs; hormonal and nutritional requirements or deficiencies vary from person to person. Whatever we choose, the fact remains: preventive measures can protect us from serious ailments.

# 2

# Medicating Symptoms Versus Addressing the Cause of Disease

*The human body is its own best apothecary . . .*
*because the most successful prescriptions*
*are those filled by the body itself.*

**Norman Cousins**

Millions of Americans are afflicted with arthritis.[1] But seldom do we see this epidemic linked to the denatured foods that are sold to us daily in almost every grocery store. The role that pasteurized and processed foods play in disease is never mentioned by advertisers, nor is the fact that we are routinely ingesting foods containing additives and preservatives.[2] The final insult to the body comes when we choose unnecessary prescription drugs over organic foods as medicine. The overuse of antibiotics, sedatives, decongestants, and antihistamines along with habitual poor food choices can create a buildup of toxins that penetrate the intestinal wall and may contribute to diseases like cancer, arthritis, and other autoimmune disorders.

We may only experience vague or minor symptoms, but if we don't heed them, their underlying cause can lead to a major disease. For instance, toxin buildup may cause an imbalance of the intestinal bacterial flora, which will eventually lead to nutrient malabsorption and a wearing down of the intestinal wall. This allows the penetration of toxins, unassimilated animal proteins, and undigested starches into the body and bloodstream—causing sluggishness, autointoxication, nutritional deficiencies, and allergies.[3] This, in turn, results in metabolic disturbances throughout the body. As we continue to overconsume enzymeless foods year after year, pathological changes will occur, especially in collagen, the connective tissue throughout the body. "The resultant accumulation of toxic wastes and mineral deposits completes the picture of a fully developed arthritis," says Dr. Paavo Airoli.[4]

Perhaps in another century, maybe sooner, the medical establishment will better understand the medicinal powers of whole, organic foods and the positive effect that natural food supplements and some herbs have on various disorders. It will be a hallmark day when all doctors recognize the importance of working in conjunction with nutritionists, chiropractors, homeopaths, acupuncturists, and other natural health care professionals. Sound too good to be true? Well, it doesn't cost us anything to hope, or to have a vision for a better tomorrow. Great changes have been born from such dreams.

## MONOPOLY IN THE HEALTH CARE SYSTEM

Today we remain far from this vision. Power and greed within the health care arena have, unfortunately, captured the control of our "free" enterprise system. Julian Whitaker, M.D., quotes from the FDA's Dietary Supplement Task Force report that one of the missions of the FDA is to "insure that the existence of dietary supplements on the market does not act as a disincentive for drug development."[5] To alleviate this problem the natural molecule is then changed by manufacturers to a synthetic molecule for a profitable form of medication.

Institutionalized medicine in the United States feels threatened by other health care professionals whose natural treatments consistently achieve permanent benefits for their patients. It's interesting to note that health care competition doesn't seem to exist in other countries where governments (such as Germany's) bear most of the cost of herbal remedies so it's naturally more economical for the government to help the patient get well as quickly and efficiently as possible. This is a great incentive for competent free enterprise medicine. Author Robert McCaleb explains it well in *The Energy Times*: Governments else-where—Europe, Canada, and the Asia—have "approved organic pre-ventive medicines aimed at reducing the risk of heart disease, liver disease and cancer."[6] With all the existing drug regulations in the United States, our ability to obtain valuable nutritional supplements, herbs, or natural hormones from a physician is severely restricted.

It's disconcerting that our free enterprise system has not found a way to make safe and effective health therapies more easily attainable so that the public could also be privy to natural forms of pain relief and healing. Unfortunately, under our present medical establishment, if a treatment is effective, but not profitable, it's unlikely that the consumer will hear about it. Yet the studies on phytonutrients and phytohormones are available, and it's worth the effort to investigate[7] and well worth our time to do our part in actively promoting natural organic foods.

## DISEASE PREVENTION AND THE USE OF MEDICINAL PLANTS

The medical field uses medication and calls it prevention because the symptoms *temporarily* diminish. Their focus is on the treatment of symp-toms, not the illness, or the ultimate cause of the disease (which con-tinues to progress). An example of this can be seen within the nervous system, which is one of the master controllers of our immune system. My personal experience was that once my nervous system was functioning without interference, my body was better able to use needed nutrients. Seen in this context, *preventing* disease goes so much further than just treating symptoms.

Preventing disorders depends on the quality of food we ingest, as well as how to combine foods for optimum assimilation and utilization. Another related principle is the complex subject of "protein" foods. Harvey and Marilyn Diamond explain that for protein to be assimilated properly it "must first be digested and split into its component amino acids. The body can then use these amino acids to construct the protein it needs. The ultimate value of a food's protein, then, lies in its amino acid composition. . . . There are no 'essential' amino acids in flesh that the animal did not derive from plants, and that humans cannot also derive from plants."[8] This essential function of amino acids, as well as many other factors, should be understood when comparing flesh protein with plant protein.

Another important consideration in the prevention of disease is nutritional supplementation.[9] Vitamins A, E, and C, selenium, zinc, manganese, acidophilus/bifidus, enzymes, and so on all aid the body in healing itself. These natural foods and supplements contain antioxidants, which fight free radicals found in the body.[10] The high temperatures used during the manufacture of processed foods tends to create free radicals. These are harmful to the body because they rob good cells of their power to continue to keep us healthy. This will be discussed in further detail in the following chapter.

Antioxidants offer protection to the body because they support the immune system. Keep in mind that the most effective, and the more impressive, results in preventing or attacking arthritis come from the natural forms of these supplements, not the synthetic forms.

## CHALLENGING CONVENTIONAL CONCEPTS

People have increasingly been pointing to the need for change. It is heartening to see that included among these people are growing numbers of medical doctors practicing natural alternatives. Perhaps, with the patient's encouragement, they will gradually limit the use of prescription drugs and begin to suggest botanical remedies in the beginning stages of illness. Some already have, and these wiser physicians will agree that healing power comes not from the physician, but from within the body.[11] The wise patient will focus on the preventive care that allows this power to work.

Alternative therapies that were controversial in the past are often seen now for what they are: fundamental to our well-being. We are gaining more confidence in natural remedies with their increased use and as more research and knowledge is obtained, we are being given the opportunity to take a personal interest in our own welfare. It's encouraging to know that researchers are making the distinction between conclusions based on nutrition and herbology studies versus conclusions drawn by food and pharmaceutical manufacturers in the interest of selling more products. The biochemists, medical doctors, and professional authors who are on the front line keep us abreast of natural alternatives. These noble souls are our future leaders in the health care industry.

## MEDICAL RESEARCH SUPPORTS NUTRITIONAL THERAPY

Alan Gaby, M.D., spent over ten thousand hours of intensive research in the "caves of medical libraries." He points out that here "much wisdom and innovation lie gathering dust." He found myriad reports documenting nutritional therapy as it is linked to the practice of medicine. He says that "virtually none of this information was taught in medical school, nor could any of it be found in standard textbooks. . . . I tried [the remedies] in my practice. . . . Most worked just as the articles said they would." In medical school Dr. Gaby was told to "shut up about that mineral and vitamin research stuff; never mind that it's published in medical journals."[12] In the end, however, Dr. Gaby prevailed; he pursued his interest in natural alternatives. He and other medical doctors continue to use these alternatives, leading the way to a healthier and more active lifestyle.

Dr. Jonathan V. Wright, another leading authority on nutritional medicine, has treated thousands of patients successfully with diet and supplements, curing them naturally of depression and insomnia. His fresh and natural approach was so effective that it began to cast suspicion on the medical establishment's widespread use of antidepressants and sleeping pills. Unfortunately, this seemed to provoke the FDA, who raided his Tahoma Medical Clinic in Kent, Washington, on May 6, 1992, taking away all his state-of-the-art diagnostic equipment, vitamins, minerals, patient charts, and educational material.[13]

This unfortunate occurrence is not uncommon, and is still happening in other areas of the country. When we hear about these ordeals, it should remind us that natural approaches that can improve the quality of our lives are worth fighting for. Fortunately, such solutions are still being pursued by innovative and courageous businesses and health professionals.

## OUR PRIORITIES: HUMAN LIFE OR SHELF LIFE?

Nutritional deficiencies are one of the main reasons degenerative diseases, such as certain types of arthritis and even cancer, are so prevalent these days. Not only is the overconsumption of food common in our society, but we also are eating foods depleted of nutritional value. Author Humbart Santillo sums it up concisely: "Today's society is overfed and undernourished."[14]

The enzymatically live ingredients that are processed out of many foods in order to extend shelf life are the very ingredients needed to improve the quality of our lives. Since the the packaged-food industry is mainly concerned with maximizing profits, the outcome for the consumer is dismal. Supplying the population with whole foods containing the necessary enzymes, vitamins, minerals, and essential fatty acids needed for healing are not high on their priorities. And the consumer pays the price.

White bread, for instance, has a long shelf life because the whole wheat "berry," the part that contains the nutrient value, or "life," has been removed. This inner berry contains the essential oil and the numerous vitamins and minerals needed by the body to function normally. Only unaltered whole food has the ability to support optimal function of the body's biological organs and provide the most complete hormonal and nutritional balance. But these crucial substances required for health are removed during processing. The manufacturer's rationale is economics. Foods will become rancid more quickly if these substances are not removed. So long shelf life becomes first priority, and the consumer is left with buying and ingesting pure starch—food that is devoid of essential vitamins and minerals.[15]

An article in *Health Freedom News*, a publication that keeps the public abreast of new research in the field of natural alternatives, reports the distressing news that "the adulteration of bread, flour and processed cereals by 'enrichment,' doubled the U.S. death rate from heart disease in only ten years."[16] Since the bleaching of flour began in 1904, this denaturing of food has become one of the causes of joint disease leading to arthritic conditions. Nothing about this process is holistic: The products are stripped of natural nutrients and then dosed with additives to make them "enriched." In other words, the live enzymes are removed and substituted with synthetic additives to preserve shelf life. *Enriched*, therefore, is a highly deceptive term.

Dr. Santillo, author of *Food Enzymes—The Missing Link to Radiant Health*, points out that undigested food "putrefies in the colon, producing by-products that are reabsorbed through the intestinal tract and deposited in the joints and tissues of the body."[17] Supplementing with enzymes, vitamins, and minerals is essential for increasing the total enzymatic activity within the body. In fact, eating plenty of raw food will also aid the digestive process.

Arthritis occurs when our organs have been overworked by years of abuse trying to cope with the foods that are now refined, overcooked, and microwaved. Dr. Santillo states, "These detrimental processes are causing dramatic changes in the food that we eat. They have rendered our foods enzyme-deficient, causing imbalances in our organs, acting as a predisposing cause of disease."[18] For instance, Dr. Julian Whitaker reports that microwaving can cause anemia by decreasing hemoglobin levels, which can in turn lead not only to thyroid dysfunction, but also to rheumatism.[19] Dr. Whitaker continues, "Researchers at Stanford University Medical Center reported that microwaving breast milk just to warm it a little destroyed 98% of its immunoglobulin-A antibodies [and] 96% of its liposome activity that inhibits bacterial growth [and that] the microwave radiation itself may have caused damage to the milk above and beyond the heating."[20]

The convenience of microwaving has robbed us of essential nutrients and lowered our immune system capabilities. Dr. Ana Sota of Tufts University warns us that ingesting food that has been microwaved in plastics can mean taking in more xenoestrogens.[21] These produce estrogen-like activity and are toxic and foreign to the body.[22]

Now let's think for a minute about what happens in our body when we don't eat raw fruits and vegetables on a regular basis. Studies have found that our digestive organs become exhausted when most of the food we eat consists of refined or fast foods. This causes the pancreas to become overactive and secrete large amounts of enzymes, which can lead to an enlargement of one or more of our vital digestive organs, such as the pancreas, the liver, and so on. Dr. Santillo explains, "An enlarged organ is often a pathological condition, showing the beginning signs of degeneration. . . . Since the enzymes in raw food actually help digest the food they are contained in, and can be absorbed into the blood and used in other metabolic processes, we can assume that taking enzymes or eating a large percentage of raw food, will help take the stress off not only the pancreas, but the entire body."[23]

This increased activity of our enzymes also occurs when we are suffering from any kind of illness or stress. Some of the enzymes we possess are superoxide dismutase (SOD), lipase, amylase, and protease; these (and others) initiate chemical reactions that allow the digestion and utilization of nutrients.[24] In acute diseases they work hard as a defense mechanism in the body. They can, therefore, be more rapidly used up during times of metabolic stress or when the body has a higher temperature than usual. This is why some natural health practitioners are recommending enzymes in place of drugs. We are now finding a definite link between a healthy immune system and our enzyme levels.[25] Enzymes are integral in circulation and thereby the relief of excess swelling and pain.[26] For this reason, they should be considered first when fighting arthritis.

## ENZYMES FROM RAW UNCOOKED FOOD

Food in its natural state—prior to being overprocessed and homogenized—could actually give us an abundance of nutrition and energy right up to old age. Dr. Francis Pottenger, a medical researcher, performed experiments in the area of pasteurization. After giving his cats a diet of pasteurized whole milk, he found that they became arthritic. The cats who drank only raw whole milk had not the least evidence of arthritis.[27] If our diet doesn't consist of raw milk and whole foods, and if the majority of our fruits and vegetables are cooked instead of raw, we are missing out on essential enzymes and amino acids. Some believe that enzyme deficiency is a "forerunner to disease."[28] Enzymes could be the medicine of the future for not only arthritis, but also cancer and many other chronic diseases.

A change of diet to include foods rich in protein from vegetable sources is beneficial for tissue growth and repair.[29] Animal protein can be taxing on the kidneys and liver because it can cause a buildup of certain toxins such as nitrogen, which may then be transformed into uric acid.[30] When too much uric acid has accumulated in the system, crystals of the substance can be deposited into the joint space, leading to a painful arthritic condition known as gout.[31] This process is further explained by Paavo O. Airola, N.D.: "toxic wastes are then deposited in the tissues and may cause autointoxication and sluggishness—the factors usually associated with development of arthritis."[32] Taking an enzyme called uricase (which is not produced by the body) has been found to be useful for the breakdown of uric acid.[33]

Diets high in protein have also been implicated in poor bone health. Excessive amounts of protein can cause the calcium reserve in the bones to be withdrawn in order to alkalinize (neutralize) the increased acidity of the blood created during the digesting of the protein. High protein consumption, regardless of how high the calcium intake is, has been shown to cause more calcium to be excreted in the urine than is absorbed by the body.[34] This same leaching of calcium also occurs in the presence of high levels of phosphoric acid from cola consumption as well as from caffeine intake[35] and smoking by-products.[36]

It is a fact that natural enzymes in our foods aid digestion. Renowned author Hanna Kroeger in her writing *God Helps Those Who Help Themselves* explains that "enzymes aid in transforming proteins into amino acids"[37]—and protein cannot function in our body unless it's broken down! Cooking food destroys approximately 85 percent of its original nutrients as well as many of its enzymes.[38] According to Dr. Santillo, after food has been subjected to high temperatures, much of the "protein has been destroyed or converted to new forms which are either not digestible by body enzymes or digested with difficulty."[39]

## THE ROLE OF ENZYMES IN ARTHRITIS

Enzyme supplementation has been used for over forty years in many European countries to control inflammation. Many clinical studies show that enzymes support the immune system by creating a beneficial response in the inflammatory process associated with arthritis.[40] Unfortunately, we don't hear much about the importance of over-the-counter enzyme therapy in the United States because prescription medications are much more familiar. However, it's hard to ignore this emerging field of immunoenzymology (the science concerned with immune reactions associated with enzymes) even though this treatment has been "administered to over 15 million patients during the past 15 years and . . . by all reports appear[s] to be safer than most other modalities of treatment currently available."[41]

One study shows enzyme formulations to be superior to orthodox antirheumatic agents because they are more efficient and lack the dangerous side effects of NSAIDs and other new-and-improved drugs.[42] The Medical Enzyme Research Institute has proved how enzymes "can be used to alleviate the symptoms of rheumatologic disorders, including . . . morning stiffness, pain, joint swelling," and of course loss of strength and flexibility.[43] Enzymes are natural biological aids that remove foreign agents found in the blood,[44] in the synovial fluid, and in the cartilage of the joints.[45]

Scientists tell us that enzyme combinations aid in various digestive activities. In other words, they are *synergistic;* they work together in various bodily processes. Taking a balanced enzyme combination is far more effective than taking just a single enzyme. For instance, pancreatin and bromelain, taken together, act as natural anti-inflammatory agents, making them effective for rheumatoid arthritis.[46] Bromelain enhances the assimilation of pancreatin, improving digestion. Papain (derived from papaya) digests not only wheat gluten, but also other proteins.[47] Protease or peptidase also function in protein breakdown. These enzymes support our immune system. Lipase, found primarily in nuts, seeds, and some fruits, breaks fats down into their simplest forms, monoglycerides and fatty acids.[48] Carbohydrate breakdown is completed by the enzyme amylase. This enzyme breaks down starch into simple sugars and subsequently into glucose.[49] Since each of these enzymes is necessary for the proper breakdown of our foods, a combination would help to reduce a buildup of toxins and subsequent deterioration of the joints.[50]

## THE POWER AND POTENTIAL IN PHYTOCHEMICALS

The more we learn about phytonutrients, the more we find they are becoming the safer and sounder means to achieving good health. These natural sources, when used appropriately against disease, can be excellent medicine. Immune system enhancers for many arthritic conditions and an incredible number of natural cancer cures exist in the form of herbs, raw foods, essential fatty acids, vitamins, minerals, antioxidants, enzymes, and plant-based hormones. All of these are available in a variety of forms without a prescription (teas, topical creams, sublingual drops, and so on) and pose no health risks.[51] This will be discussed further in chapter 3.

Many former arthritis patients have become natural health care enthusiasts as a result of their own positive experience with unconventional arthritic treatments—the kinds that focus on detoxifying the body, reinforcing the immune system, balancing body chemistry, and stimulating the metabolism. In fact, grave or fatal diseases like cancer and arthritis have been cured by combining a detoxing program with complementary medicines found in phytochemicals.[52]

## ROOT CAUSES OF ALLERGIES AND ARTHRITIS

It is important to recognize the similarity of all the various forms of arthritis, rather than stressing their differences. Some of the direct and indirect causes of arthritic conditions are allergies, genetic predispositions, endocrine factors, stress, and biomechanical and neurological dysfunction. But one of the major contributing causes may be a poorly functioning gastrointestinal tract. Poor nutrition and candida overgrowth eventually cause excessive permeability in the walls of the intestines, creating a "leaky gut" syndrome. As a result, larger proteins are able to enter the bloodstream without being digested, which can create allergy-type symptoms. Research confirms a definite correlation between food allergies and arthritis and rheumatism;[53] the patient's allergies were reduced, so were the symptoms of rheumatism and osteoarthritis.[54]

A variety of foods can directly or indirectly aid in joint health. But they cannot work properly if the patient suffers from associated food allergies. It is important to first check for such allergies and avoid these foods that are highly allergenic: Common villains are beef, pork, milk products, eggs, shellfish, wheat, citrus juices, nuts, chocolate, and coffee. Other problem foods include bacon, baked goods, beef tallow, bouillon cubes, cake mixes, candy, canned foods, crackers, dairy substitutes (powdered milk or egg substitutes), fatty meats, hot dogs, packaged cold cuts, margarine, mayonnaise, monosodium glutamate (MSG), refined rice, saccharin, aspartame (seen on labels as NutraSweet), salad dressing, sausage, smoked foods, and foods made with white sugar.[55]

Joint inflammation may also be brought on by ordinary foods eaten in excess, or by an unusual food eaten for the first time. Joint pain and swelling may be manifested immediately or may take as long as several days after a food is ingested. Immediate symptoms may indicate some type of allergy or food sensitivity. But how are chronic symptoms that are caused by allergies detected?

An IgG4 food panel test is a blood test that can reveal a delayed adverse response to foods ingested at any point during one's life. It is a reliable test and may be covered under insurance. Since common foods and foods we crave are often the culprit of joint inflammation and chronic conditions, the IgG4 test is highly recommended. Unfortunately most medical doctors are not trained in the specialty of nutritional health and are therefore not aware of the purpose and importance of this test, let alone that it exists. Instead, an IgE test is typically ordered. This test only indicates immediate allergy symptoms and can often produce false-positive results. The cause of long-term chronic conditions will often not be shown by this test.

Another cause of rheumatoid arthritis is a persistent bacterial infection in the digestive tract. Even such substances as the casein in milk or gluten in breads (both of these are proteins) can have systemic inflammatory effects.[56] When we consume an overabundance of gluten-rich foods on a regular basis, it can gradually form a heavy coat of mucus in the small intestine. This inhibits the villi (fingerlike projections on the wall of the small intestine) from absorbing nutrients from partially digested food. Over time this will interfere with the digestion and assimilation of our food.[57] Gluten-rich grains can also have a detrimental effect on the myelin sheath, the outer coating of the nerves. This may be the cause of multiple disorders that have gone undetected for many years.[58] Fortunately, many health food stores now carry gluten-free products such as gluten-free pizza, bread, pasta, cereal, and bagels. I've also been told that if you cook the dough well or toast your bread when making sandwiches, it's possible the gluten will be cooked out of it.

And although lectin, another protein found in plants, can be useful in defending the plant against predators, it can also instigate systemic inflammatory problems in humans if their lymphoid tissue in the gut is hypersensitive to it.[59] Considering these causes, it's understandable why people find that their chronic inflammatory disorders improve after fasting.[60]

The overconsumption of acidic foods is also related to the development of arthritis and osteoporosis. Believe it or not, too much protein (with the exception of green-leaf protein) is a main culprit. This is because it increases the acidity of our blood. Although protein is important, arthritis and osteoporosis can develop if one eats too much acidic food such as meat and cheese (with the exception of cottage cheese), instead of alkaline foods such as barley grass, carrot, apple juice, and other fruits and vegetables.[61]  *eat these*

reasons

Sir W. Arbuthnot Lane, a nutritional authority and eminent surgeon in Britain, supports this theory. He believes that some "forms of rheumatism are due to the disturbance of the acid-alkaline balance." He tells us that the predisposition to rheumatism in some people "can only be successfully countered by a diet which puts all its emphasis upon alkaline-forming foods."[62] Arthritis, regardless of the type, is symptomatic of a much more serious underlying problem that generally affects the entire body. Arthritic symptoms are sometimes a cry for nutritional help.

Another way to protect our body from toxic buildup and help it heal itself is by combining foods properly. According to Harvey and Marilyn Diamond in *Fit for Life*, combining foods from our established food pyramid philosophy does not work in practice and has created many digestive problems.[63] Observe the results of such a diet by looking around you. People are more overweight and unhealthier than they've ever been. One of the reasons for this is that combining starches with protein causes chemical incompatibility within the body.[64] We need to learn about food combining that will help the digestive tract do its primary job of detoxifying the body—not creating the ill effects of chemical imbalance.

Antacids wouldn't be a household item and would most likely come off the shelf if we better understood how demanding it is on the digestive system to eat meat and potatoes in the same meal. Ingesting protein with any starchy food, whether rice, noodles, or bread, will generate an acidic toxin in the body that produces fermentation, heartburn, and acid indigestion. This has been known since 1945 when Arthur Cason, M.D., did experiments showing that "eating protein and carbohydrates at the same meal retards and even prevents digestion."[65] Dr. Herbert Shelton's Health School also found and taught that protein could not be properly digested when eaten in conjunction with starchy foods.[66]

The Diamonds say that if you're going to eat flesh food you should combine the meat with "high-water-content food" such as salads and

51

lightly steamed vegetables. The latter foods aid in optimum digestion because they can break down in either an alkaline or acid medium.[67] If you want a potato, serve it as the entree with steamed vegetables and a salad. You can even add butter or cheese. This type of combining aids in digestion, assists those interested in losing weight naturally, and conserves energy needed for the body to detoxify.

We might want to take notice of the powerfully strong and healthy animals that live in the wild. They instinctively stay away from mixed fare. Animals are either vegetarian or carnivorous and don't depend on antacids.

## THE NEED FOR LIFESTYLE CHANGES

Author Judy Lindberg McFarland says it well: "When our food is hydrogenated, homogenized, refined, microwaved, preserved, emulsified, pasteurized, chemicallized, colored, bleached, and sterilized, something is lost. In many cases, it is *health* that is lost!"[68] And because of all the denaturing of foods, it is imperative for us to make dietary changes to clear out the toxic residues that have accumulated in our cells after many years of drug therapy or ingesting unhealthy chemicals from food, water, and the air we breathe. Once the body has been detoxified, it's amazing how the cells in our bodies more efficiently utilize clean air, organic raw food, and natural vitamins (preferably in capsule form instead of tablets) and minerals (preferably in liquid form).

I was not aware of these choices in my youth, and my own body eventually became a fertile ground for arthritis, strokes, and other physical disabilities. I finally realized the power of consuming enzymatically live foods when I changed my diet and began having more energy and strength. Author Helen Macfarlane explains that unless we eat wholesome foods and take food supplements and antioxidants on a regular basis, "dietary deficiencies may result and these can play a large part in the onset of illnesses such as rheumatism and arthritis."[69]

It is no mystery that arthritis rates are rising as a result of lifetime exposure to the wrong diet, excessive environmental estrogens (xenoestrogens), and prescriptions of additional synthetic estrogens as well as anti-inflammatory drugs used in lieu of natural alternatives. The creation of new and wondrous medicine often stifles true advancement and innovation—and, what is worse, ignores the power within all of God's pharmacy.[70]

## FRESH FROM THE GARDEN

Each of us carries our own healer within. Our body works better when we fuel it properly, particularly when we consume fresh, whole foods. We should be more concerned than ever about knowing how long it has been from the time foods have been picked to the time they are actually sold in the store. It is usually a lot longer than we think! Who knows how long a food has been frozen or intensely heated, or to what extent it has been processed before it gets to our dining-room table? Many of the real nutrients and phytohormones that can create an ideal physiological balance may have been lost.

Dr. Santillo sheds further light on this subject, suggesting that purchasing organic food and spending our precious time destroying most of the nutrients by cooking it is "poor economy and unsound ecology."[71] Ninety-year-old marathon runner and former World Senior Boxing Champion Noel Johnson is a prime example of the payoffs of good eating habits and a wellness-oriented lifestyle. His adage is: "If you have to cook it, overlook it." This may not always be possible, but raw or *very lightly cooked* (when necessary) foods should be our mainstay. Elizabeth Baker was diagnosed with two incurable conditions— cancer and Addison's disease. Now in her 80s, she is living proof that, with perseverance and discipline, life-threatening diseases can be turned into a life of health and energy. She strongly believes "raw, living foods have an abundance of oxygen. They also have all other nutrients necessary to be effectively utilized by the body." We don't get enough oxygen in our "oxygen-poor world," she says, and we need to make up for this by breathing in fresh air as often as possible. "Degenerative disease proliferates where cells don't get oxygen." Baker continues to explain that, according to cell biologists, "if cells get enough oxygen, they cannot become cancerous," and that cooked and refined or processed foods have no oxygen. Most problems are caused or made worse by poor eating habits.[72]

## DIETS ARE EASY; THE MANAGEMENT IS HARD

Any diet requires modifying habits and developing a good deal of restraint. Old habits die hard. For instance, it takes a great deal of effort to read what's actually in the packaged food you want to buy. It's handy to have a magnifying glass to read the list of ingredients, usually on the back. You won't need glasses to read the label on the front; it's always in large print. But, of course, you won't get a whole lot of useful information from this advertising either.

It takes a conscious effort to change from overprocessed and overcooked foods, and to substitute copious amounts of pure water for drinks that are high in processed sugar, caffeine, artificial coloring, and preservatives—products that are high in calories but low in nutritional value.

The primary source of our vitamins and minerals should always be, of course, high-quality fresh foods, preferably grown organically. Buy vitamins from a health food store that contain "whole food" ingredients and not the synthetic substitutes commonly found in grocery and drugstore supplements. These substitutes are foreign substances that cannot be properly metabolized by the body and can eventually cause toxic buildup.[73] For more information on food sources for all vitamins read *The Real Truth About Vitamins and Antioxidants* by Judith A. DeCava, M.S., L.N.C.

When ill or in pain, try a change of routine. Instead of going to the medicine cabinet for a painkiller, antacid, or anti-inflammatory drug, search for healing remedies in the health food stores or grocery stores that specialize in organic foods. When it comes to arthritis, keep in mind our previous discussion in chapter 1 about the toxicity that occurs and builds up in the body after taking pain relievers and anti-inflammatory drugs (NSAIDs). Sol Grazi, M.D., provides many more studies that clearly demonstrate their long-term serious consequences, not only causing liver and kidney damage, but cartilage damage, which ultimately leads to joint degeneration.[74] If you have taken medication for a long period, it has possibly altered your gastrointestinal system's ability to absorb nutrients.[75] Also, as Jeffrey S. Bland, Ph.D., points out, arthritis or inflammation is not just a "localized phenomenon"; it's a systemic condition.[76] Therefore, any form of arthritis or other inflammatory disease may require going beyond the orthodox approach. You may need a treatment for the whole body, not just the localized pain. And, of course, individual bodies differ depending on how well one's immune, endocrine, and neurological systems are functioning.

In looking to the causes of arthritis, many researchers have focused on the connection between intestinal flora and lymphocyte activity. Dr. Bland states, "The intestine is generally recognized as the largest lymphoid organ in the body, encompassing the greatest number of lymphocytes and generating almost 70 percent of the antibodies."[77] As an immune system response, these lymphocytes are directed toward lymph nodes, mucosal lymphoid organs, and inflamed joints.[78]

So we need to restore normal bacterial flora in the gastrointestinal tract and look for foods, including fiber, that will cleanse our bodies before rebuilding. For example, kefir, a form of fermented milk, cleanses the digestive tract of harmful microorganisms (including parasites and disease-causing yeast and bacteria) and produces a light mucous coating that encourages the colonization of healthful bacteria. It normalizes the pH of both the intestinal tract and the blood. Organic kefir improves digestion and immunity and provides complete protein and important minerals, such as the B vitamins, and even vitamin K.[79]

Some authorities consider kefir superior to yogurt. It is more digestible, and the milk does not require heating as in yogurt culture. It may be easily cultured on your kitchen counter from grains you can reuse indefinitely (obtainable by calling 1-888-KEFIR-4U). Any milk, including rice milk or coconut milk, may be used, although whole raw cow's milk or goat's milk is ideal. A freshly made batch will have the most active cultures. As a bonus for the lactose intolerant, the bacteria and yeast present consume most of the lactose in the fermentation process, and the lactase (an enzyme) should eliminate any lactose that remains.[80] For more on this nutritious food, you might enjoy reading Donna Gates's *The Magic of Kefir.*

## SYSTEMIC POISONS  *Flouride*

The importance of drinking *pure*, preferably distilled, water cannot be overemphasized. The chemicals in tap water such as chlorine and fluoride are damaging to connective tissue. There is conclusive evidence that "fluoride is accelerating the breakdown of collagen."[81] This causes a wide assortment of bone problems.[82] In fact, thorough testing has shown fluoride to increase the incidence of fractures because it creates an inferior quality of bone mass.[83] Fluoride is a toxic by-product of aluminum and phosphate fertilizer. It is also a potent enzyme inhibitor causing not only gastrointestinal inflammation, but also pathological changes in bone leading to a significant risk for bone fracture.[84] On top of everything else, fluoride negatively affects the thyroid gland. In fact, the book *Prescription for Nutritional Healing* cautions us to avoid products that contain flouride. "Chlorine and flouride block iodine receptors in the thyroid gland, resulting in reduced iodine-containing hormone production and, finally, in hypothyroidism."[85]

What's frightening is that chlorine and fluoride are added to our drinking water and many people don't realize the effects: muscle weakness, nausea, abdominal cramps, tremors, hypotension, and even respiratory failure.[86] Drs. James and Phyllis Balch warn "The poisonous substance that fluoride is derived from, builds up in the body, causing irreparable harm to the immune system."[87] If you live in a city where your tap water contains fluoride, it is highly recommended that you buy distilled water or use a reverse osmosis system.[88]

You may also want to consider fluoride-free toothpaste, which can be obtained in health stores. For many decades it has been known that supplemental fluoride can alter the structure of tooth enamel leading to decay. It is also an enzyme inhibitor—enzymes that are needed for digestion. John R. Lee, M.D., found that fluoride has been categorized with cyanide in the textbooks on toxicology and is considered a "potent enzyme inhibitor."[89] It's no wonder inflammatory diseases are so prevalent in today's society, given that chlorine and pesticides are also found in our tap water. These factors, along with our prescribed medications, are major obstacles in our effort to restore our body to homeostasis.

## SUSTAINING THE INNATE FORCE

For those who are insured, it's much easier and more economical to go to a family physician for health problems such as allergies, digestive disorders, and so on than it is to change their lifestyle. But down the road it's more taxing on the body. Prescribed drugs can often lead to blood cell abnormalities, clots, liver disease, or even death.[90]

The more we begin to understand what the body needs, the more we can support its marvelous design for using natural foods to cleanse and regenerate tissue. When we do, we should begin to see changes in our health—from a state of infirmity to one of vitality. And this can happen through choosing foods with ample amounts of antioxidants, vitamins, minerals, and enzymes, as well as drinking plenty of *pure* water and keeping up with a regular program of exercise. A sensible and complete turnabout in routine can influence almost everything we do, think, and feel.

So, before considering yet another drug for a condition that is still festering, why not take advantage of the unadulterated forms of healing that powerfully address the cause of disease? Already present in creation are curative substances that will help us achieve optimal energy and make us less vulnerable to the effects of environmental stress. This personal effort will also affect much more than just our physical health.

*Your choice of diet can influence your long-term health prospects more than any other action you might take.*
**Former Surgeon General C. Everett Koop**

# Part II

# Study the Cure
# Before Treating
# the Pain

# The Healing Power of Natural Substances

*Minerals, vitamins, proteins, chlorophyll and enzymes are the keys to health. Together, they maintain our cells . . . and work to correct any abnormal condition that occurs . . . serv[ing] to invigorate natural activities within the body.*

**Yoshihide Hagiwara, M.D.**

While the wrong diet can trigger the inflammatory cycle, the right diet can help to detoxify and cleanse the body, which in the long run can fight inflammation and disease.[1] An increasing number of doctors are beginning to recognize the correlation between what we eat and the health we enjoy, and our diet's role in stimulating balance and homeostasis. Dr. Barbara Joseph is an obstetrician and gynecologist, as well as a survivor of breast cancer. She shares with us what she learned the hard way: "We need to buy and eat organic food whenever possible. This nourishes us, keeps carcinogenic chemicals out of the body and at the same time makes a powerful political and economic statement. Health is not achieved by going for yearly checkups, getting Pap tests or scheduling mammograms."[2] She goes on to tell us that good health depends on how we live—our lifestyle and the food choices we make.

And the true staff of life is raw and unprocessed food. Is it also a vital factor in combating arthritis? That's a thought-provoking question. Let's examine some of the remarkable natural food sources that are available to help, but seldom used by the millions of patients afflicted with immune deficiency disorders. We can start with a single vegetable, cabbage, and use it to illustrate the life force within natural foods. Did you know that a daily intake of *sulforaphane* and *indoles*, as found in cabbage, broccoli, and other cruciferous vegetables, can help prevent disease?[3]

Raw cabbage is a remarkable vegetable. It can serve as a blood purifier and it is therapeutic for conditions such as gout, rheumatism, cancer, and many other diseases, says A. M. Liebstein, M.D.[4] Unfortunately, when you cook it, things change. In the process of being cooked, cabbage loses many of its minerals and most of its powerful medicinal effect. Bruce Berkowsky, Ph.D., states "Green cabbage (having a higher nutrient content and being more active medicinally [than red cabbage]) . . . is a remarkably potent remedial entity, being a specific treatment for many cases of arthritis, gastrointestinal ulceration, skin eruption and various metabolic imbalances, including those characterized by obesity. . . . The indoles contained within fresh raw cabbage also neutralize metabolic toxins. And because of the high fiber and potent antioxidant content (vitamins A and C) it is "equally responsible for its anti-cancer properties." Dr. Berkowsky continues, "according to researcher Durk Pearson, cabbage stimulates a liver enzyme system which inhibits the activity of carcinogens."[5]

Just substitute cabbage for lettuce in your salad, and you've taken a significant step toward better health. Dr. Kurt Donsbach, a leading nutritionist, recommends mixing it with raw potato, carrots, cauliflower, sprouts, celery, and tomatoes for a healthy meal. I have always found cabbage to be a great staple. And it stores better than lettuce, for longer periods—which makes it useful to take on those extended camping trips.

Dr. Allan H. Conney, director of the Laboratory for Cancer

Research at Rutgers University, found that rosemary, curcumin (an agent responsible for the anti-inflammatory action of turmeric),[6] and green tea all suppress cancer growth. They do so, according to Dr. Conney, by "acting as antioxidants, neutralizing free radicals before they reach the cell's kingpin, DNA."[7] In simple terms, free radicals are unstable molecules that are produced in the body as a result of environmental or dietary toxins (tobacco smoke, X rays, car exhaust, rancid fats, preservatives, and so on). They can damage the cell membrane and genetic material.[8] They can also create joint inflammation. Green tea has been shown to have anti-inflammatory properties, as well as gastrointestinal healing effects that facilitate digestion.[9] Following are some specific foods that have been found to be particularly helpful for arthritis treatment and prevention.

## A POTPOURRI OF CURES

### Cayenne

The active ingredient in hot peppers is capsaicin. It's rich in vitamin C and A—both wonderful antioxidants. A variety of studies have shown that after only two weeks of rubbing cayenne cream on the area of sore joints four times a day, "80 percent of subjects with osteo- or rheumatoid arthritis benefitted" from the treatment.[10] The consumption of cayenne also aids in decreasing the swelling and pain associated with arthritis.[11] Biochemists at the Central Food Technological Research Institute in Mysore, India, discovered that red pepper and capsaicin are beneficial in lowering cholesterol levels, and that capsaicin overpowered the harmful effect of fatty foods.[12]

### Cherries

Cherries contain flavonoids that have "anti-inflammatory powers, free radical scavenging and the ability to strengthen cartilage, tendons and joints."[13] Compounds such as anthocyanins and proanthocyanins found in most dark red and blue berries have a remarkable ability to strengthen collagen. Eating at least half a pound of cherries (one cup) a day will cause a significant reduction in uric acid, often preventing gout and other forms of arthritis.[14] Making cherries part of your diet may be an excellent therapy for this painful disease.

## Potassium

Eating foods that contain a good supply of potassium is important for a healthy nervous system. Potassium is an anticalcification mineral: It aids in preventing calcium from depositing in the joints, which can cause stiffness.[15] Potassium also inhibits sodium retention, and potassium bicarbonate reportedly improves our calcium-phosphorus balance and reduces bone loss.[16] Bananas and lady's mantle are rich in potassium.[17] Foods with potassium-related medicinal benefits include green leafy vegetables, wheat germ, kelp, blackstrap molasses, fresh sesame seeds, salmon, and sardines. James and Phyllis Balch's *Prescription for Nutritional Healing* lists foods such as brown rice, brewer's yeast, garlic, winter squash, nuts, figs, dates, raisins, wheat bran, and yams as foods that promote potassium-related healing.[18]

Paul and Patricia Bragg tell us of the healthy form of potassium that's in vinegar. Two teaspoons of organic apple cider vinegar will fight the buildup of acid crystals that have a tendency to form in our body over the years. These eventually cause disorders such as bursitis and other joint problems.[19] Add a small amount of honey or pure maple syrup for palatability.

## Sea Salt versus Table Salt

Why should we insist on natural unrefined sea salt instead of refined table salt? First of all, we need to understand what *refined* means. Author Jacques de Langre explains in *Seasalt's Hidden Powers* that during the processing of table salt, all of the healthy trace minerals are removed.

Sulfur, magnesium, calcium, potassium, and iodine are just a few of the numerous macrominerals that are purged. These important ingredients are extracted from the salt and are then separately packaged as "essential minerals" and sold to the food industry. Table salt is also treated with commercial bleaching agents. The whiteness you see as you sprinkle it on your food by no means denotes purity. It's just been bleached. More important, chemically treated salt doesn't unite as easily with human body fluids.

This refined table salt is laden with additives and is one of the reasons we experience water retention, back pain, and even kidney problems. Refined salt does not permit liquids to freely cross body membranes and blood vessel walls. The accumulation of fluids eventually creates stagnation in the joints, leading to edema and inflammation.

Unprocessed sea salt, on the other hand, provides us with a balanced array of many essential minerals that are not abundant in the plant world. Dr. de Langre states, "Salt is the single element required for the proper breakdown of plant carbohydrates into usable and assimilable human food. Only when salt is added to fruits and vegetables can saliva and gastric secretions readily break down the fibrous store of carbohydrates."

Natural sodium is vital to "restoring digestion; relieving allergies, and skin diseases; and preventing many forms of cancer." Dr. de Langre also writes that natural sun-dried sea salt provides our cells with increased energy and permeability; aids in metabolism, muscle contractibility, and nerve function; and provides resistance to bacterial infections. The body, however, cannot use the so-called pure refinement of salt. Dr. de Langre points out, "It is no coincidence that the amniotic fluid that bathes the human embryo is salty and grey like the ocean from which all life on this planet has issued forth." He further explains that most healing salts consist of over seventy "noble minerals" of the sea.

Lastly, a high-quality salt contains the precise amount of magnesium salts needed to remove sodium chloride from the body after the salt has performed its countless medicinal functions. Magnesium salts in microdosages ($^3/_4$ of 1 percent) are essential in breaking down nutrients, regulating bone development, dissolving calcium deposits, and preventing kidney stones. Dr. de Langre reports that "magnesium salts, along with other precious trace elements, allow a thorough elimination of toxins while effectively flushing the body of excess sodium and calcium."[20] For more information on sea salt, contact the Grain and Salt Society, 273 Fairway Dr., Asheville, NC 28805, 800-867-7258.

## THE WONDERS OF VITAMIN B COMPLEX AND VITAMIN C

Many arthritics have abnormally low levels of vitamin B complex and vitamin C in their bodies. Restoring these to normal with the appropriate supplements will rebuild collagen and "stimulate . . . adrenal glands to produce more cortisone,"[21] which reduces inflammation. The use of B complex has been shown to actually reverse degeneration in joints. According to Stuart Berger, M.D., 100 mg per day is effective and quite safe.[22]

E. C. Barton-Wright and W. A. Elliot, physicians at the Rheumatic Clinic in London, discovered that when patients were orally given pantothenic acid (one of the B complex vitamins), osteo- and rheumatoid arthritis improved.[23] Many of us have diets extremely deficient in pantothenic acid. Doctors believe that highly processed foods are one of the main reasons rheumatism is so prevalent in the Western world. Dr. Roger J. Williams says it's very possible that those who suffer from a variety of arthritic conditions could achieve permanent, rather than temporary, results through proper nutrition and joint manipulation.[24]

Dr. Williams also stresses the body's need for not only pantothenic acid, but also B complex, vitamins A and C, magnesium, calcium, phosphorus, and other minerals. These vitamins and minerals are necessary to "feed adequately the cells that are involved in keeping the bones, joints and muscles in healthy condition."[25] Another B vitamin, niacinamide, has also been effective in treating osteoarthritis. Dr. William Kaufman, a nutrition specialist, uses approximately 100–150 mg for his patients, whereas Dr. Donsbach found that as much as 500 mg may be considerably more effective.[26] A pilot study showed niacinamide to have a positive effect on the synovial fluid, which in turn could aid in cartilage repair.[27]

Because vitamin C (always with bioflavonoids) is so important in building up the immune system, it significantly aids in the prevention of arthritis. It has an important role in the formation of collagen and wound healing.[28] Further studies show that vitamin C aids in cartilage health and is beneficial for those afflicted with osteoarthritis.[29] This is because it can repair cartilage tissue and is a cofactor in protein synthesis. Norman Shealy suggests 2 g per day for both osteoarthritis and rheumatoid arthritis.[30] And James S. Gordon says that 3–6 g per day for rheumatoid arthritis stimulates natural anti-inflammatory responses.[31]

As long ago as 1930 it was discovered that rheumatoid disease was related to a deficiency in ascorbic acid, or vitamin C. In fact, one physician, Dr. Robert Cathcart of Los Angeles, found that vitamin C was crucial in treating arthritis, lupus, and other autoimmune diseases. This assumes, of course, that it is used in combination with a good diet and other healthy treatments.[32]

## OTHER ESSENTIAL VITAMINS, MINERALS, AND NUTRIENTS FOR NERVES, MUSCLES, AND BONES

Some authorities maintain that we need at least 2 to $2\frac{1}{2}$ times as much dietary calcium as phosphorus.[33] The recommended dietary allowances (RDAs) for adults (which are in the process of being revised) list the calcium-phosphorus ratio as approximately 1:1.[34] However, this amount of phosphorus seems too high, based on several other studies.

An excess of phosphorus can create a calcium deficiency by binding calcium in the gut and rendering it useless. Too much phosphorus can also bind up other important minerals.[35] Studies reported in the *Journal of Nutrition* show that high intakes of phosphorus may overstimulate the parathyroid gland, promote bone loss, impair synthesis of the active form of vitamin D, and disturb calcium balance, especially in menopausal women.[36] Such an altered calcium-phosphorus ratio in the body will interfere with the ideal chemical balance needed for bone health.

Some of the foods that cause this mineral imbalance are found in abundance within the typical American diet (high-protein foods, sodas, caffeine, alcohol, table salt, and so on). In processed foods there is also widespread use of phosphate additives (orthophosphates, polysulfates, pyrophosphates), which can create a phosphorus overload that further disrupts the body's chemistry.[37]

Nancy Appleton, Ph.D., warns that "if functioning calcium is lacking in the blood, it will actually be removed from the bones and may be deposited in the weak joints."[38] These hard calcifications (which constitute osteoarthritis) cause crippling pain and inflammation. Arthritis patients have discovered that after fasting for several days on distilled mineral water the arthritis pain often clears up. (This natural therapy is not suggested for patients who are currently on medications requiring food for proper administration.)[39]

Finding a supplement that will fortify our body with the perfect ratio of minerals is a challenge. First of all, we know that phosphorus aids in bone formation as long as it's in the proper proportion with calcium and other minerals. Eighty percent of phosphorus used in our body is in our bones and teeth; and the rest is found in our nerve and muscle tissue.[40] So, if we're going to supplement, an appropriate ratio is essential.

James and Phyllis Balch affirm in *Prescription for Nutritional Healing* that "a proper balance of magnesium, calcium and phosphorus should be maintained at all times,"[41] along with the various other minerals and vitamins that are needed for their assimilation.[42] Dr. Appleton also emphasizes that all minerals "work in relation to each other."[43] In her book *Lick the Sugar Habit*, she states, when "phosphorus decreases, functioning calcium also decreases."[44] She further explains that if one's calcium intake is increased without a change in the phosphorus level, the surplus calcium can become toxic.[45]

Researchers have also found that sucrose and refined carbohydrates will dilute the necessary minerals found in food.[46] They will also alter the calcium-phosphorus ratio in the blood.[47] In other words, high glucose ingestion reduces calcium resorption by the kidneys and increases its urinary excretion. This in turn interferes with mineral metabolism,[48] and it can create a secondary magnesium deficiency, eventually affecting the health of bone.[49] It's quite clear that magnesium plays a vital role throughout the body as an important enzyme catalyst. It assists in calcium and potassium uptake.[50]

Minerals and vitamins perform synergistically with one another.[51] They "work as catalysts, promoting the absorption and assimilation of other vitamins and minerals [and] this is why taking a single vitamin or mineral may be ineffective, or even dangerous."[52] Dr. Appleton stresses the importance of getting our calcium from the right foods rather than from calcium supplements.[53]

Other reports say that the glorification of calcium by the dairy industry is a hoax on the American people. Would we do better to take magnesium rather than calcium supplements? High-calcium and low-magnesium intakes are contributing to an acceleration of arthritis, diabetes, heart disease, and even senility.[54]

Alan Gaby, M.D., mentions that other minerals and vitamins such as zinc, copper, silicon, boron, manganese, vitamin K, and certain fatty acids are also needed in their proper balance for optimum calcium assimilation.[55] Vitamins A, C, D, and F are also required in their proper balance.[56] These cocatalysts work to help us avoid arthritic conditions such as calcification of tissues, including bone spurs.

Today we find magnesium to be an essential partner with calcium.[57] We are also discovering that stress, brought on by drugs or physical or emotional strain, depletes magnesium. Because of these factors, some practitioners are recommending an even higher magnesium-calcium ratio. Dr. Gaby, in his book *Preventing and Reversing Osteoporosis*, states that there was a "dramatic improvement in bone mass" when prescribing 600 mg of magnesium and 500 mg of calcium.[58] When Dr. Gaby put his patients on 800 mg of magnesium and only 400 mg of calcium, he also witnessed improvement in women who suffered from premenstrual syndrome.[59]

All this has made me focus on the likelihood that, in addition to osteoporosis, joint disorders such as temporomandibular joint (TMJ) syndrome and bone spurs might be exacerbated by a mineral imbalance. Indeed, Dr. Appleton says that such an imbalance can even cause arthritis, kidney stones, gallstones, and other disorders.[60] Incidentally, since many trace minerals can be toxic in nonphysiological doses, a natural source, such as sea vegetation, is desirable.

There are seventeen minerals that Dr. Appleton calls "essential in human nutrition. If there is a shortage of just one of these," she writes, "the balance of activity in the entire system can be thrown off." Such deficiency can have a negative impact, causing other nutrients to become "ineffective and useless."[61] Dr. Appleton advises maintaining a 2.5:1 calcium-phosphorus ratio for optimal health and recommends home testing to monitor both your calcium-phosphorus balance and your pH level. (For information on how to obtain a home test kit contact Nancy Appleton, Ph.D., P.O. Box 3083, Santa Monica, CA 90403.)

Vitamin D plays an essential role in keeping the "serum calcium and phosphorus concentrations within the normal range."[62] Vitamin D also promotes mineralization and thus strengthens the skeletal bones.[63] We shouldn't depend on our foods to provide vitamin D because most foods do not include this vitamin. Exposure to sunlight provides this critical vitamin needed by the body.[64] Being out in the sun for just fifteen minutes a day has been known to relieve arthritis pain.[65] People who don't get enough sunlight have been found to often be deficient in vitamin D. *The Arthritis Bible* reports that "men and women need 400 IUs per day. This dose equals the U.S. RDA for people under 50, and it is double the U.S. RDA for people over 50."[66]

Wheat germ, vitamin E, and vitamin A are also included in the many nutrients that can improve the usefulness of calcium.[67] Vitamin E is essential to neuromuscular health. It is important, though, to be aware that there are differences between the natural and the synthetic form of these vitamins. The chemical and molecular distillation process to which vegetable oils are subjected when they are transformed into synthetic vitamins prior to being put into a pill does little to enhance them for human consumption. Learn to read the labels. Synthetic vitamin E, which is biologically ineffective, will list "dl-alpha tocopherol" in its ingredients. Natural vitamin E will list "d-alpha tocopherol" on its label. This natural vitamin E is utilized properly by the body.[68]

Be cautious too when buying vitamin A and avoid the synthetic forms, which include retinoic acid, isotretinoin, accutane, and beta-carotene.[69] In its natural form, vitamin A supports the immune system and helps the body attack bacteria and viruses. "We need to incorporate into modern medicine God's antibiotics, against which bacteria does not develop a resistance," says Julian Whitaker.[70] One good source of vitamins A and D is halibut liver oil. (See appendix A for sources.) Other good sources of vitamin A that has been converted from beta-carotene are animal products such as butter and eggs. Eating a variety of fruits, vegetables (especially yellow ones), and wheat germ may be the best way to supplement a carotene complex.

Wheat germ oil has also proven to be successful as long as it remains stable and is not heat processed. Once it becomes unstable, wheat germ oil can become rancid by oxidation.[71] Dr. P. Vogt-Moeler's research has shown that wheat germ has many biologically active ingredients, in addition to tocopherols, which provide beneficial effects.[72]

## GARLIC, ONIONS, AND HERBS COMBAT ARTHRITIS

Rheumatism and osteoarthritis can be caused by a hidden virus.[73] The best-known natural antiviral and antibiotic agents are contained in garlic and vitamin C. Garlic contains a biologically active compound called allicin. This sulfur alloy is activated when whole fresh garlic is cut, crushed, or chewed. Clinical studies of garlic's antibacterial properties have found it to be "effective against a variety of bacteria, including *Streptococcus*, *Salmonella enteritidis*, and *Staphylococcus aureus*, and even some known to be resistant to antibiotics." A crude extract of garlic can be more effective that most antibiotics.[74] Stephen T. Sinatra, M.D., in his book *Optimum Health* speaks about garlic's ability to reduce swelling through its anti-inflammatory effects.[75]

Garlic has also been proven to be beneficial for osteoarthritis and gout. Onion, a cousin to garlic, has similar effects, although to a lesser extent.[76] A combination of herbs and plants such as yellow dock, yucca, black walnut leaves, wormwood, and fenugreek seed are also effective in clearing out the damage done by certain viruses.[77]

## ARTHRITIS—A DIETARY CAUSE

Arthritis can be linked to a combination of factors, causing a variance in symptoms from one person to another. But the stronger our immune system, the better our chances of fighting arthritic diseases. Fresh fruits and vegetables (rich in enzymes, vitamins, and minerals) help build up our immunity. They are the "antioxidant powerhouses" that can help protect us from developing arthritis, as well as other diseases. We greatly increase our chances for good health when we eat plenty of fruits and vegetables; they contain the fiber that cleanses the body and is basic for good health.[78]

On the other hand, certain factors may weaken our defenses. Processed sugar is enemy number one, and it is ubiquitous. It's used in virtually all packaged foods, fast foods, and soft drinks. Dr. Gaby reports that consuming refined sugar decreases the capability of some of the white blood cells (neutrophils) to expel bacteria.[79] Sugar not only suppresses the immune system; it also depletes the body and creates many other undesirable conditions: "Since refined sugar contains virtually no vitamins or minerals at all, it dilutes our nutrient intake, resulting in an across-the-board 19% reduction in all vitamins and minerals in our diet. Thus, because of our high intake of sugar we are getting less magnesium, folic acid, vitamin $B_6$, zinc, copper, manganese and other nutrients that play a role in maintaining healthy bones."[80] When reaching for that donut, pastry, candy bar, or other sugar-coated food, think about the rock candy experiment from grade school in which a mixture of sugar and water was suspended on a string: "The sugar crystals precipitate [collect] onto the string (fun on a string—not so much fun in a blood vessel)."[81]

In the book *There Is a Cure for Arthritis*, Paavo O. Airola, N.D., identifies all foods made with white sugar as the first and foremost destroyers of health.[82] White sugar and white flour are simply "devitalized" carbohydrates.[83] They have been stripped of their nutritional value. Sugar also affects the body in a multitude of adverse ways— from degrading the health of the bones to destroying the regularity of monthly menstruation.

When treating diseases such as arthritis, it's important to look at factors that create imbalance and toxicity. When Dr. Donden, a Tibetan doctor, was asked about American food, he said he thought it tasted very good, but that sugar is used like salt. It's in everything— even hot pepper sauce. Dallas Clouatre, Ph.D., argues that sugar "will induce cold diseases, such as diabetes, as well as rheumatism; it will also make great problems in old age."[84]

And what are most Americans eating when they need an energy boost? Maybe they reach for a cola (12 oz has 12 teaspoons of sugar) or binge on ice cream (1 cup contains 7 teaspoons of sugar). Just one slice of apple pie contains 15 teaspoons of sugar, and when our children eat sugar-coated cereals having 8 teaspoons of sugar per cup, it's no wonder they show hyperactive behavior. Elaine Newkirk, N.D., writes that variations in blood sugars can cause tantrums when the blood sugar is high and depression when the levels drop.[85]

Meanwhile, what is sugar doing to the rest of our body? Some of our chronic disorders may be nothing more than a simple allergy to an overabundance of sugar.

Sugar is in almost everything we eat, from luncheon meat to canned foods. Sugar can be listed on labels as sucrose, glucose, fructose, dextrose, honey, and syrups, including high fructose corn syrup, or HFCS, which is highly allergenic. We've discussed how high amounts of consumed sugar can eventually cause calcium-phosphorus imbalance. Eliminating some of these foods from our diet will be one step in maintaining a proper calcium-phosphorus balance and in turn avoiding degenerative joint disease.[86]

And since we're on the subject of sugar, don't be tempted by words like *sugar-free*. It's better to read the label carefully before jumping from the frying pan into the fire by adopting sugar substitutes like NutraSweet (aspartame). Woodrow C. Monte, Ph.D., Director of the Food Science and Nutrition Laboratory at Arizona State University, tells us that "when aspartame is metabolized, it releases methyl alcohol (wood alcohol), a known toxin that is highly dangerous to humans." Dr. Monte warns us that "once in your cells, methyl alcohol converts to formaldehyde, a cancer-causing agent.[87] G. R. Austin, Ph.D., gives us the alarming news that "Methyl alcohol is used as a polar solvent for plastics, paints, and varnishes; as an antifreeze; and in the manufacture of formaldehyde . . . Methyl alcohol has a selective action on the optic nerve and can cause blindness."[88]

Even the disease lupus has been associated with the use of Nutra-Sweet. Dennis W. Remington, M.D., tells us that "large doses of aspartame change the ratio of amino acids in the bloodstream and the balance of various neurochemicals in the brain."[89] So now we're finding the use of aspartame may be one of the many major factors that's linked to autoimmune diseases such as multiple sclerosis and lupus.[90]

What's more, aspartame is a toxin that stimulates the brain while at the same time damaging nerve cells by blocking the energy the cells need to function.[91] Details of the bittersweet truth about aspartame can be pursued further in the publications listed in appendix B.

If you really need a sweet taste in your foods or drinks, try an unrefined, safer, and healthier substitute called *stevia*.[92] Dr. Daniel B. Mowrey's investigation into herbal remedies has led him to write about their scientific validation in healing.[93] It turns out that stevia not only sweetens our food but is also used for medicinal purposes in other parts of the world. In Paraguay, for instance, it helps conditions such as hypoglycemia by nourishing the pancreas and helping in its ability to function normally.[94] Tests have shown that the plant's sweetening agent, the glycoside stevioside, is 300 times as sweet as granulated table sugar. But stevioside is potentially far more than a nonfattening sugar substitute: it actually triggers hypoglycemic activity, reducing blood sugar levels as it sweetens. Hence it can be a true lifesaver for many diabetics."[95] Check it out at your local health food store. Bake and cook with it and know that, when you crave something sweet, stevia is actually nutritious.

Previously, we discussed how food allergies and refined carbohydrates may be a major contributor to arthritis symptoms. On the other hand, some foods combat arthritis. These are chiefly whole-grain cereals, whole-grain breads, and brown rice.[96] Essential nutrients contained within whole plants such as alfalfa are calcium, iron, magnesium, choline, phosphorus, potassium, sulfur, protein, the amino acid tryptophan, and all the vitamins, including K.[97] Other literature stresses molasses, and of course fresh, organic fruits and vegetables.[98] Alfalfa is a wonderful food for relieving arthritis, as are dates, wheat germ, kefir, and food sources of germanium. These sources can include garlic, shiitake mushrooms, onions, aloe vera, comfrey, ginseng, and suma.[99]

## NUTRITIONAL BALANCE

Joel Robbins, M.D., is a naturopath, chiropractor, and well-known lecturer on the secrets of good health. The simplicity of his explanation is powerful. If only putting the solution into practice could be as simple! Dr. Robbins suggests that approximately 80 percent of our diet should consist of alkaline foods. In other words, we should eat more fruits, vegetables, almonds (for a good balance of minerals and for bone building),[100] and whole grains (unprocessed foods that contain live enzymes) while consuming only 20 percent acidic foods, which include dairy products, meat, enriched grains (bleached white flour), and cooked foods. He says it's unfortunate that most of the foods we consume, such as sugar, salt, coffee, tea, and processed or refined foods, are also acidic; it means that the amount of acidic foods we eat will almost always rise much higher than the recommended 20 percent. But if we can keep the alkaline foods to around 80 percent, we will consume enough nutrients to keep the body well and to neutralize the 20 percent acidic foods we often wish to consume. So we don't have to give up meat and other foods entirely if we take into consideration this ratio.[101]

Dr. Robbins stresses that this pH balance is one of the most important factors in maintaining health and life. He says that when the alkaline percentage goes below 80 percent there's not enough vitamins and minerals, and vitamins and minerals are the catalysts that keep the cells healthy. The pH imbalance will cause the body to search for nutrients elsewhere. In the end the body compensates for this lack and starts robbing minerals from other areas, such as the cartilage, tendons, ligaments, and bones in order to obtain nutrients for the cells and neutralize this acidic condition. An alkaline-acid imbalance can be a large factor in the onset of arthritis, osteoporosis, and other diseases.

And as our cells become more acidic they become less efficient and thus unhealthy, leading to a condition that your doctor may diagnose as "just getting old." When our body is in this acidic state, and we continue to introduce more acidic foods, they will be treated by the body as toxins. Allergies, joint problems, and other diseases will manifest themselves. Simply put, a *toxin* is defined by Dr. Robbins as "a substance that the body has no use for whatsoever, and will cost the body energy and nutrition to deal with it."[102] Let's look at one of the all-too-common joint abnormalities that can occur as we age.

When people find calcified knobs or bone spurs on their joints they often think it's because they have too much calcium and so they begin to avoid it. But according to Bernard Jensen, Ph.D., author of *Arthritis, Rheumatism and Osteoporosis: An Effective Program for Correction through Nutrition*, even in these cases our bodies require calcium, which is found in a variety of wholesome foods. If supplemental calcium is needed, Dr. Jensen suggests bonemeal, which is considered a whole food because it's made up of joint material, the material that is needed to replace our degenerative joints. When you provide the body with something it already has, it naturally will be drawn to it. This is the homeopathic principle "like attracts like."[103]

Dr. Jensen also tells us that we need "to have enough sodium [not table salt] to balance the calcium, so it doesn't come out of solution and deposit in the joints." He continues that sodium from the right foods "softens any hard material . . . and keeps the body limber." Dr. Jensen says that those who suffer from back or arthritis problems require more sodium than the average person. This is because sodium aids in neutralizing the pH balance. The best form of calcium and sodium is found not in supplements, but in foods, where it is in a bio-organic form. Arthritics may do better consuming foods that are higher in this mineral in an effort to reverse the problems associated with this disease. Whey is very high in sodium. Additionally, butter, swiss cheese, celery, swiss chard, brown rice, pineapple, and squash also contain sodium.

Here again we find that the body becomes sensitive when the blood is very alkaline or is very acidic. If the majority of our diet consists of acidic foods, our elimination channels can't work well and we will feel it in our joints. The outcome is often enlarged joints and even spurs.

## MYTHS ABOUT NIGHTSHADE PLANTS AND RHEUMATISM

There continues to be quite a controversy about nightshade plants and arthritis. Some authors tell us that since the tomato is a member of the nightshade family, it is a prime instigator of arthritis. Other authors, like Jean Carper, say there is no substantial evidence for this.[104] Jason Theodosakis, M.D., argues that "although there are many claims that removing nightshades will cure arthritis, no scientific proof has been offered."[105]

So consider, then, one nightshade plant: the eggplant. The eggplant has a reputation for possibly being able to protect arteries from cholesterol abuse. In Nigeria it is thought to protect against rheumatism; and in Korea, the dried plant is applied topically to the painful joint to cure rheumatism. Austrian scientist Dr. G. H. A. Mitscheck found that eating eggplant with a high-fat, high-cholesterol meal releases a chemical that binds up the fat in the intestines so it will not be absorbed into the bloodstream. Serendipitously, it seems to "help cancel some of the ill effects of the cheese in a dish like eggplant parmigiana."[106]

And remember the days when people suffering from joint pain put a raw potato (another nightshade plant) in the pockets of the clothes they were wearing in order to thwart rheumatism? Hot potato water was even applied locally to relieve gout, lumbago, and other problems.[107]

There may be some merit in the charges against nightshade plants, however. Every body is different and some immune systems just will not tolerate these vegetables because of the alkaloids in the plants. Alkaloids may accumulate in tissue and build up slowly over time, creating allergy symptoms. For some this will be manifested as poor vision, dry eyes, depression, constipation, slow urination, and even swelling and painful joints. Foods considered to be in the nightshade family include potatoes, tomatoes, tobacco, eggplant, peppers, modified food starches, and some spices.[108]

If you suspect that one or more of these plants is the cause of arthritis symptoms, eliminate them for at least three months and monitor the results. It's important to heed the signs of your own body when making food choices. When I first began exhibiting arthritis symptoms, I left nightshade foods out of my diet. For me it did not solve the problem, but for others it might be a solution.

## JUICING

Juicing is an economical way to obtain nutrients directly from food and an efficient way to provide nourishment to our cells. For instance, the juice of certain vegetables such as onions, garlic, tomatoes, and radishes has a natural antibiotic effect. Paavo Airola, N.D., writes that "cucumber and onion juices contain hormones needed by the cells of the pancreas in order to produce insulin."[109]

Books that were extremely helpful to me in learning the importance of juicing were *Fresh Vegetable and Fruit Juices* by N. W. Walker, D.Sc., and *There Is a Cure for Arthritis* by Paavo O. Airola, N.D. They explain that there is a real connection between the food we eat and the debilitating pain of osteoarthritis. As we learn from *The Arthritis Cure*, "Certain foods can help stem the destruction of joints, while others may help to ease the pain or prevent the problem in the first place."[110]

Juicing also stimulates enzymes to protect the cells from oxidation. Juice "fasting" (avoiding solid foods) clears out whatever toxins (uric acid, metabolic and calcium deposits) have built up from years of eating refined foods. It helps to prevent cancer, allergies, and heart and inflammatory diseases.[111] This natural therapy even stimulates growth hormones, which normally decline with age.[112]

If you're considering this therapeutic regime and suffer from any chronic or debilitating conditions, educate yourself thoroughly on all aspects of juice fasting; and in cases of such conditions, it might be wise to be under the supervision of a doctor who specializes in nutritional healing. For excellent books on the topic of nutritional healing, please see appendix B.

It may be most useful to obtain our juices primarily from vegetables, because fruit juice contains a higher concentration of sugar. Some nutritionists suggest diluting juice with distilled water when first adding juice to one's diet. This helps control glucose and insulin levels, which is essential in the management of inflammatory diseases (connective tissue and intestinal disorders, diabetes, asthma, and allergies, to name a few).[113] It's also important to use *organic* raw fruits or vegetables (free of pesticides, herbicides, and so on).

Juicing works because the living nutrients in the fruits and vegetables get into the bloodstream and down to the cellular level immediately. The body does not have to expend energy or time to process food through the whole digestive system.[114] The body can then immediately experience the power of these intact raw foods that are rich in complete forms of vitamins, minerals, and phytochemicals (indoles, isoflavones, polyphenols, saponins, and many more).

When arthritis pain hits, it's frightening; and most people will do whatever it takes to get back to a normal pain-free existence. That's when I began juicing and first experienced its medicinal power. Using the regimen outlined below eased my arthritic discomforts significantly. And it got me back on a healthy course. I could feel the difference in a few days, but continued on for another week until I regained my strength. Each person's schedule differs and each case of arthritis requires a personal approach.

### Early morning

Freshly squeezed grapefruit juice (grapefruit's salicylic acid helps dissolve abnormal calcium buildup and the accumulation of foreign matter). Shake well with one tablespoon of halibut-liver or cod-liver oil (contain omega-3 fatty acids, which subdue inflammation, and provides vitamin D, necessary for calcium absorption).[115]

Midmorning

Blend kefir with a tablespoon of brewer's yeast (good for the health of the eyes),[116] juice a favorite green vegetable, or take barley green and alfalfa (best source of absorbable calcium). If you're still hungry after several hours, eat apples, grapes, or a banana.

Noon

Juice: celery including the stalks and leaves for complete nutritional value. (Celery's sodium helps maintain the calcium. It's also a natural diuretic.)[117]

1:00 P.M.

Juice: carrots and spinach. (This combination aids the blood and lymphatic system in carrying away waste matter while nourishing the nerves and muscles of the intestines.)

2:00 P.M.

Juice: carrots and celery. (This combination rebuilds and regenerates the cartilage and joints.)

3:00 P.M.

Juice: carrots, beets, and cucumber (enzyme support; stimulates the liver).

4:00 P.M.

Juice: carrots, celery (antirheumatic agent used in Australia),[118] parsley, and spinach (rich in chlorophyll).

5:00 P.M.

Juice: carrots, spinach, turnip, and watercress.

7:00 P.M.

Eat a wholesome supper.

For optimal nutritional benefits, drink the juice immediately after it's been prepared. Also, remember to consume about a gallon of distilled water every day. Some patients have relieved their arthritis by consuming carrot juice exclusively; some have had success with distilled-water fasts and homemade vegetable broth (not derived from cubes) or soups. Frequently people get relief within weeks. In other cases, when there has been many years of toxin buildup and damage to the joints, you may feel worse before you feel better. The detoxing process may take more time to restore health. Discipline, consistency, and time are key factors in achieving success.

Some folks would rather not take on all this responsibility, not to mention all the work. They'd prefer to be under the direction of a professional. And that's understandable, as breaking old habits can be quite a chore; and ill health may make a juicing program difficult to manage. Those working outside the home may just not have the time or effort required. If this is the case, you could consider joining one of the many biological clinics or spas that provide therapies to treat arthritis. They have had wonderful results in strengthening the immune system, restoring the body's healing power, and making arthritis a condition of the past. The health professionals at these centers are helpful in directing and motivating proper diet and exercise.

You'll find that some of the health spas give organic apple cider vinegar and honey drinks with a meal. This compensates for an insufficient release of hydrochloric acid, and it aids in digestion. (A wet pack of apple cider vinegar can be also placed directly on a painful joint to relieve the discomfort.) If necessary, or preferred, they will substitute fresh lemon, apple, or pineapple juice for vinegar. Incidently, pineapple contains enzymes for protein breakdown and is an excellent source of bromelain, which contribute to its anti-inflammatory effects.[119] Papain, from papaya, reduces inflammation and destroys bacteria associated with stomach disorders. Lemon and grapefruit also "have a neutralizing effect on the body acids,"[120] making them potential medicines for arthritic conditions. Professionals as well as laypeople are now recognizing the importance of juicing. Author N. W. Walker, D.Sc., finds "thousands the world over have testified with gratitude to the benefits derived from fresh raw vegetable juice.[121] In his book he explains how specific combinations of fresh juice will aid the body in detoxing and healing specific ailments. People have been cured from a variety of diseases when they began juicing organic fruits and vegetables, stories of which are recorded in *Alternative Medicine*, by the Burton Goldberg Group.[122]

The degree to which we improve our diet will also be the degree to which our organs will function more efficiently and our inflammatory disorders will come under control. An improved lifestyle that embraces preventive medicine can bring multiple benefits to all our physical and mental functions.[123]

Whichever changes you decide to make, over time you can actually acquire beneficial results. Whatever you choose, it's important that you enjoy the juice you're going to be drinking habitually. And remember that over time we actually acquire a taste for foods we previously didn't enjoy, especially as we realize the health benefits they bestow. As the "body is a living organism made up of living cells," it continually requires living or raw food to persist at peak performance.[124]

As strength and energy are regained (which could be days for some people and perhaps months for others), fresh raw fruits and vegetables, multigrain foods, and homemade vegetable broth may be introduced during the day. Excellent foods such as brown rice mixed with wheat germ, brewer's yeast (which provides B complex vitamins), and blackstrap molasses with pecans, walnuts, or sunflower seeds sprinkled on top can relieve the pain associated with rheumatoid arthritis. Fresh nuts and seeds are essential. A combination of pineapple and cottage cheese is also excellent for the relief of arthritis.[125]

Not having the time or the means to enjoy the luxury of a health spa, I had to put together my own regimen. Initially, I was quite disciplined about juicing, but I must admit my schedule didn't always allow me to do it as much as I'd like. That's when I began incorporating a green barley drink into my daily routine. One teaspoon a day helped immensely. This natural, organic food was invented by Yoshihide Hagiwara, M.D., a research pharmacologist. It contains lightweight protein molecules that are fully utilized by the body. It's a better and more usable source of protein than the protein provided by meat. It also contains sixteen different vitamins, eighteen amino acids, twenty-five minerals, enzymes, chlorophyll, and so much more.[126]

If you are a meat eater, purchase meat products that are free of synthetic growth hormones and antibiotics. See appendix A for a listing of some of those who produce such meat and poultry. Ask your grocery store to carry meat from one of these or other free-range or organic meat producers. Synthetic growth hormones and antibiotics can cause serious hormonal imbalance when they accumulate in the body and disrupt the endocrine system by blocking receptor sites.[127] And fighting to achieve hormonal and nutritional balance by choosing live foods that help the regeneration of our cells is the single most important step in preventing arthritis.

Once on the mend it's a good idea to juice once a day, or perhaps once a week or month, depending on your health, time, and personal preference, in addition to eating wholesome foods. This gives the body a chance to rest and rid itself of accumulated wastes. Meat eaters should limit their consumption to small portions three times a week. Too much meat "is known to produce uric acid, one of the main culprits in engendering and fostering arthritis."[128]

## HERBAL REMEDIES FROM NATURE'S APOTHECARY

Since the beginning of time, herbal remedies have been high on the list of alternative medicines. Herbs come in a variety of forms such as capsules, liquid extracts, teas, flowers, aromas, creams, and even powders (used for making poultices). There are many books (see appendix B) that explain which herbs are beneficial for specific conditions, and how and when to use them. Such information combined with a knowledgeable resource person can lead you in the right direction.

Herbs can be sprinkled over hot foods or salad or infused as teas. Green tea provides an immune system boost in the morning. Teas labeled "detox" or "fasting" contain herbs used to cleanse the digestive system and rid the body of environmental toxins. During a stressful day licorice tea (good for the adrenals) made with pure water is helpful. I like to add a few drops of cayenne and ginger (both are good for arthritis problems). This combination also keeps the digestive system healthy.

Nighttime teas containing a combination of herbs such as chamomile flowers, passion flower, spearmint leaves, lemongrass, catnip, and hops are excellent for calming the nerves and aiding in restful sleep. During sleep, tissue regeneration and optimal healing take place. Sleep is medicine, although the role of sleep in healing arthritis is often neglected.

Remember that herbs may affect different people in different ways depending on their symptoms and needs. In other words, you may find one combination of herbal remedies to be helpful, while another person may discover that a different blend of herbs may produce the best results, even if both of you have the same symptoms of arthritis.

Herbs also work better when used in conjunction with natural food and plenty of pure water fortified with liquid minerals. Herbs often work more efficiently when used together, especially when symptoms are interrelated. Linda Rector-Page, N.D., Ph.D., explains that some herbs have anti-inflammatory or antibiotic properties and others contain tissue-strengthening agents. It's also interesting to learn that herbs work best when used only on an as-needed basis, unlike vitamins, which should be taken daily.[129]

## HERBS FOR ARTHRITIS

Herbal remedies have been found to be extremely effective in treating joint problems and other degenerative diseases. This being the case, why isn't this information more readily available to the public? Most blame goes to the large pharmaceutical companies and their interminable advertising. They will usually ignore herbal medicines that have traditionally kept people well for thousands of years. These treasures, as well as the benefits from vitamins, minerals, and amino acids, have also been downplayed."[130]

The following are some of the major and more popular herbs that are used for arthritis. Space precludes an exhaustive discussion of dosages and potential contraindications, so I suggest that you consult a qualified naturopathic physician or herbalist to discuss your particular health issues and determine what herb, or combination of herbs, may work best for you. Be sure to let them know what other prescription drugs or supplements you are taking. Because herbs are powerful medicines, self-medication with unfamiliar herbs is not a good idea. I recommend reading Steven Foster's *101 Medicinal Herbs: An Illustrated Guide* along with the other books and studies listed in appendix B under "Vitamins and Herb Supplements."

### *Bilberry* (Vaccinium myrtillus)

The active polyphenol in this plant is called anthocyanin *(anthocyanoside)*, and it is what accounts for its luscious blue color. Many use bilberry as a therapeutic agent for their eyes, but it is much more than that. It also enhances tissue strength of other structures throughout the body. Anthocyanins fasten to collagenous structures, resulting in anti-inflammatory and capillary protection.[131]

### *Boswella* (Boswella serrata)

Boswella is a resin from a tree and is also known as *Indian frankincense*. It is a wonderful arthritis remedy; it has been found to be effective in low-back pain, osteoarthritis, rheumatism, and fibromyalgia. Boswella inhibits leukotriene production, a chemical that causes inflammation by producing free radicals. Dr. E. W. McDonagh, an osteopath in Kansas City, found boswella to be successful in treating hundreds of his arthritis patients, as their degenerative joint problems (foot, knee, ankle, and sciatica pain) cleared up. Boswella improves the circulation, promotes repair of blood vessels, and can restore the integrity of weakened joints.[132]

Some patients have found that within two to four weeks of taking boswella their pain disappeared. Like many other herbs, boswella does not produce any adverse side effects, which are frequently experienced with the use of anti-inflammatory drugs. Studies confirm that, when taken in proper doses, this botanical is safe and quite effective in fighting inflammation.[133]

## Cat's Claw (Una de gato)

*Una de gato* is becoming more and more popular because of its effectiveness in fighting arthritis, as well as other diseases. This herb is used to relieve inflammation.[134] It has proved to be more therapeutic than some other powerful herbs, such as goldenseal, echinacea, astragalus, and eleuthero (Siberian ginseng).[135] It prevents arthritis and other inflammatory disease by detoxifying and cleansing the intestines.[136] It exhibits "powerful antiviral, antimutagenic, antioxidant, and digestive-enhancing properties."[137] Components such as alkaloids, saponins, flavonoids, gallic and ellagic acid, beta-sitosterol, catechins, hyperin, proanthocyanidins, and even rutin all contribute to its effectiveness.[138] Other reports confirm that these phytochemicals (polyphenols, triterpenes, stigmasterols, campesterols, and especially isoteropodine) contribute to the enhancement of one's immune system by attacking harmful microorganisms. Quinovic acid glycosides within this herb protect the body from viruses.[139] Researchers stress that the "whole" is greater than any isolated part of this plant in providing these remarkable benefits.[140] This powerful herbal remedy should be in everyone's medicine cabinet.

## Devil's Claw (Harpagophytum procumbens)

Some arthritis patients showed a remarkable decrease in joint swelling when they used devil's claw.[141] One of the most useful effects of devil's claw is in lowering uric acid levels, which can cause painful arthritic symptoms in the joints.[142] In some countries, such as England, for example, devil's claw is sold regularly for aching limbs and inflammation associated with rheumatoid arthritis and osteoarthritis.[143] There is a case of a ten-year-old girl who had been crippled with rheumatoid arthritis for seven years. After six weeks of taking devil's claw she was finally able to enjoy her childhood. She became active in biking and skating for the first time in her life.[144] This herb's active ingredients—glycosides, stigmasterols, fatty acids, beta-sitosterols, and others—account for its anti-inflammatory and pain-relieving effects.[145]

## Ginger (Zingiber officinale)

This root is an effective antioxidant—a natural antibiotic. It is also rich in niacin and vitamin A. The herb turmeric (*Curcuma longa*—curcumin), which is in the ginger family, is known for its antirheumatic activity.[146] Ginger mends joints, inhibits pain-producing prostaglandins, and works as an anti-inflammatory.[147] Clinical studies report that patients have received more relief from pain, swelling, and stiffness from taking ginger than from synthetic NSAIDs.[148] Even better, ginger has been shown to have no side effects.[149] A mixture of gingerroot and hot water placed on a cloth can be used as a compress to pull toxins out of the body.[150] It is great to ingest daily as a hot tea.[151]

## Noni (Morinda citrifolia)

This therapeutic herb comes under a variety of names, depending on which country it's grown in. Because it has alkaloid properties and is a source of vitamin C, it has the ability to reduce inflammation and fight pain.[152] It can also stimulate cell regeneration and clean out the intestinal tract and colon—without causing the harsh side effects of dangerous drugs.[153] Its antioxidant effect fights free radical formation, which then enables T cells to aid the immune system in fighting disease.[154]

Every part of this tropical plant is used for medicinal purposes and is treasured by the Hawaiian and Tahitian people in treating common ailments such as fever and asthma. It is even used in healing wounds by applying a mixture of the plant extract with coconut oil. This precious botanical has been found to be especially useful in treating joint disorders related to arthritis.[155]

A common occurrence with certain types of arthritic conditions is the inability to properly digest and thus absorb protein foods. This can eventually cause crystal-like deposits to form in the joints. The *Morinda citrifolia* fruit can augment enzymatic function, which aids in protein digestion.[156] Because of its role in promoting enzyme action, it can help to prevent this crystalline buildup. It is suggested taking noni on an empty stomach since it will be destroyed during the digestion process while acids and enzymes are at work.[157]

## White Willow Bark (Salix alba)

Years before aspirin was introduced, patients would drink willow bark tea to relieve pain, headaches, and fever. Willow bark contains acetylsalicylic acid, the active ingredient in aspirin, and it provides a phytotherapeutic effect.[158] Today, unfortunately, the general populace uses aspirin, despite its known side effects (stomach ulcers, heartburn, nausea, and thinning of the blood).[159]

Since millions of arthritics now take aspirin daily for pain and its anti-inflammatory effect, some comments on the consequences of its long-range use are warranted here. The stomach irritation and blood thinning caused by aspirin can substantially increase one's chances of a fatal hemorrhage.[160] Furthermore, buffered aspirin reduces the formation of new bone due to the aluminum, and this accelerates bone loss.[161]

The editors of *Consumer Guide* magazine caution that many of the anti-inflammatory drugs on the market, including aspirin, can cause bloating, constipation, diarrhea, difficulty in sleeping, dizziness, headache, loss of appetite, nervousness, unusual sweating, or vomiting.[162] Many people treat fever with aspirin, but as Andrew Weil, M.D., advises, "Unless fever is dangerously high (105°F or 40.5°C), such action is probably unwise. There is clear experimental evidence that fever helps the body fight infection and that artificial lowering of fever gives invading germs an edge."[163] White willow could be advantageous since it has both antiseptic and anti-inflammatory properties, allowing the body to naturally reduce fever.[164] Some patients who don't want the adverse effects of aspirin have switched to this safer botanical. In fact, the German government has found this herb to be effective for the above conditions as well as rheumatic disorders.[165]

## *Yucca* (Yucca schidigera)

Yucca "acts as a blood purifier" and is an effective remedy for arthritis, osteoporosis, and inflammatory disorders.[166] Its effect is much like that of cortisone.[167] Robert Bingham, M.D., Medical Director at the Desert Arthritis and Medical Clinic in California, found that the use of the desert yucca plant was excellent for reducing infection and inflammation. Growing numbers of physicians are now using this with great success and have found no side effects.[168] Some clinics often prescribe that the yucca root be cut up and placed in water and "used as soap . . . or added to shampoo.[169]

## *Other Botanical Remedies for Arthritic Symptoms*

Following is an additional listing of herbs and botanicals that can ease specific conditions related to arthritis.

Bromelain;[170] turmeric;[171] witch hazel;[172] black current seed;[173]

evening primrose; feverfew;[174] yellow clover; and red clover may all be taken to relieve joint inflammation and pain.

Joint mobility and strength can be aided by alfalfa; kelp (also an excellent source of iodine and excellent for the eyes[175] and thyroid gland[176]); dandelion root (increases uric acid excretion);[177] neem leaf; prickly ash; grapeseed extract; turmeric root (quiets swollen joints and protects the liver;[178] and sarsaparilla.

For joint and muscle pain, relief can be found with the use of burdock root; capsicum;[179] blessed thistle; St. John's wort; black cohosh; stinging nettle (which can also increase circulation in the joints);[180] and meadowsweet.

Other healing botanicals that can relieve arthritic symptoms include wintergreen; myrrh; shiitake mushroom (contains lentinam, the polysaccharide "that bolsters body defenses [and]. . . autoimmune conditions");[181] yellow dock (mix with lime juice and apply to inflamed joints);[182] oat straw (calcium enhancer); aloe vera (for joint swelling and stiffness);[183] chickweed; ginkgo; chaparral leaves; comfrey; and valerian root.

Quite a few of the phytochemicals found in these herbs can also be found in fresh, organically grown fruits and vegetables. For more information, refer to "Juicing" on page 78.

## A HOMEOPATHIC APPROACH TO ARTHRITIS TREATMENT

Herbal remedies may also include homeopathic sources, which are forms of natural substances that can heal without dangerous side effects. Homeopathic medicine, founded by Samuel Hahnemann in 1790, addresses the needs of those who prefer using gentler remedies that focus on the cause of their symptoms. Homeopathic treatments are designed to stimulate the body's innate forces to act against disease. This safe alternative to the standard drug approach is a practice that, although not new, has been newly discovered and has stirred much interest in recent years. Homeopathic remedies have proved to be effective at relieving disorders due to their ability to remove deep-seated toxins from the body.[184]

In homeopathic care, minute doses of medicines of vegetable and mineral origin are given to the patient. This follows the "law of similars," first discovered by Hahnemann, who demonstrated that while a specific dilution of a substance may cause illness in a healthy person, it will remove the illness in an unhealthy person. He found that small doses were more effective, especially when they were properly diluted. The body is therefore not assaulted with larger amounts than it can handle.[185]

Hahnemann, having grown concerned over the toxic drugs associated with the conventional medicine of his day, coined the term *allopathy* to refer to traditional Western medicine. During the course of his work, he was immersed in the philosophy of a religious man, Emanuel Swedenborg, who was a student of science and believed that there was a spiritual reality more important than the natural reality.[186] This convinced Hahnemann that inner healing comes from God and that the physician's role was just to gently encourage nature to do the mending. The principles of homeopathic medicine grew out of his convictions and his research.

Controlled experiments have shown homeopathic medicine to restrain viral activity in organic tissue. During the disastrous epidemic of cholera in 1954, the death rate within the traditional medical hospitals was 50 percent, while in homeopathic hospitals it was only 16.4 percent. Certain homeopathic remedies can also be used along with allopathic medicines to combat the side effects of drugs.[187]

People are becoming aware of the importance of increasing the body's natural resistance to disease. Many health food stores, churches, and bookstores are supporting this awareness by holding seminars on how to use homeopathic remedies. Some useful reading to begin your venture in learning about homeopathy can be found in appendix B.

## FINDING THE REMEDY RIGHT FOR YOU

Finding the right homeopathic remedy can be challenging because two people with similar symptoms may be helped by completely different remedies. Below you will find a variety of remedies suitable for specific arthritic complaints. While these are available without prescription in potencies that are perfectly safe for home use, you may experience much better results if you consult a homeopath. A trained homeopath will spend time talking with you about your physical and emotional well-being and then choose the proper remedy based on your personal health history.

If you decide to experiment on your own, begin with the lower potency remedies (labeled 6 x or 6 c). Rinse your mouth and do not eat or drink anything for about 30 minutes before or after treatment. You should also avoid caffeine (no black tea, coffee, chocolate, or cola) and peppermint while treating yourself homeopathically because they tend to reduce overall effectiveness.

### Joint Inflammation and Pain Relief

arsenicum album

baptisia

bryonia

apis mellifica

podophyllum

symphytum officinalis

tabacum

iris

althaea

juglans

verbascum

lycopodium clavatum

rhododendron chrysanthum

ledum palustre

colchicum autummal

pulsatilla

calcarea carbonica

symphytum

hekla lava

lappa

juniperus

phyto-lacca decandra

salix alba

## Joint Mobility and Strength:

silicea

## Joint and Muscle Pain Relief:

| | |
|---|---|
| ruta graveolens | belladonna aurum muriaticum |
| cimicifuga | mercurius |
| arnica (oral) | silicea |
| arnica causticum (for external use) | dulcamara |
| rhus toxicodendron | |

# FIGHT FOR NATURAL WAYS TO HEAL: A BATTLE YOU CAN'T LOSE

When we're young, we think we'll continue to stay healthy regardless of the fast foods we consume, the medications we take, or the toxins we place in our bodies. And in our youth, for a time, we can get away with this abuse. But the longer we wait, the greater the possibility for disorders—for problems that ultimately end up in our joints, causing degenerative arthritis and other diseases. But why wait for this to occur when you can reestablish balance at deeper levels within the body? And why wait if you already have the ammunition to protect yourself?

Nutritionist Paavo Airola tells us that "nutrition is singularly the most important factor affecting health and disease."[188] One of the reasons nutrition is such a controversial subject is that it lends itself to fads and trends. It is not always easy to sift through what is true and what is fallacy. New scientific research continues to add to our need to challenge preconceived ideas, for instance, the establishment doctrine that cholesterol is always something to avoid. To the same degree that we need food in its natural state, we need better facts about various foods and fats.

In spite of the unconscionable bias toward natural alternatives, we are still free to act on what we now know the body needs in order to correct a vitamin or mineral or enzyme deficiency. Arthritis is a disease that can be cured, though the discipline involved can make it difficult. But when the pain is gone and the healing begins, we can finally sense a bit of triumph in mastering the existing limitations that keep disease flourishing.

So how much responsibility are we willing to take concerning health matters? It might be considered a priority since it's really up to us to reshape the prevailing attitude of masking one's symptoms to an attitude of seeking the *cause*. Furthermore, the quality of one's life, the entire life, from now to the very end of it, depends on our daily choices. There will come a day when the serenity we all hope to experience at the time of our death is as valuable to us as any other experience in our life.

# 4

# The Fat/Oil/ Cholesterol Debate

*Just as we need good quality proteins,*
*carbohydrates, vitamins, and minerals,*
*we also need good quality fats and oils*
*for physical and mental health.*

**John Finnegan, N.D.**

A recent news forecast on health issues reported that people seem to be getting fatter. This is surprising because food labels increasingly use catchwords like *fat free* and *light* (or *lite*) to describe their contents. We are also witnessing "an unprecedented rise of diseases that have never before existed"[1] despite all the foods labeled *cholesterol free*. Unfortunately, this often causes confusion and fear about what to eat. The strong influence of advertising by food manufacturers and the drug companies via the media can lead us into making poor selections—choices that contribute to disease.

It can be shown that chronic diseases often result from imbalances in body chemistry. Much of this can be traced to diet, with fats and oils being part of the problem. The subject of fat metabolism is extremely complex; and as research continues the commonly accepted theories of today may be discredited tomorrow. In the meantime we can expect more controversy, giving us all the more reason to continue searching for valid answers to help concerned consumers.

When we search for answers, it is important to know who sponsored the research (article, study) before we draw conclusions. Is a vested interest involved? Is it a pharmaceutical company or a food manufacturer that wants us to use its product? It's important, therefore, that we gain an understanding of fats and oils to assist in our interpretation of contradictory studies. Not all fats are created equal, and not all fats are bad. This chapter will discuss studies that show how some specific fats actually may help to fight osteoarthritis and rheumatoid arthritis when ingested in their *unrefined*, stable form.

## FATS COME IN MANY FORMS

John Finnegan, N.D., says in his book *The Facts About Fats: A Consumer's Guide to Good Oils* that the information we are getting on fats and oils may well be the most outrageous scandal of misinformation and greed imposed on the American public.[2] The use of polyunsaturated oils (nontropical oils that are liquid at room temperature) have intrinsically harmful properties.[3] Our higher body temperature causes these colder-climate oils (regardless of whether they are processed or not) to become rancid when ingested. These are the oils that are extracted from plants such as corn, soybean, safflower, sesame, sunflower, and peanut.[4]

When polyunsaturated oils are predominant in our diet (even in an unrefined form), or when we use commercially processed salad oil, mayonnaise, or common oil-based skin lotions (which can be absorbed), the toxic fatty acid molecules contained in them will eventually interfere with our natural detoxification process in the liver.[5] This can intensify arthritic and other degenerative diseases.[6] Manufacturers of unsaturated oils encourage consumers and fast-food restaurants to use their products by offering low prices and discount coupons. But an overuse of this type of oil often leads to an increased load of polyunsaturated fatty acids, creating the production of free radicals (unstable molecules). Udo Erasmus, author of *Fats that Heal, Fats that Kill*, discusses similar findings. Oils that are high in polyunsaturates can lower cholesterol somewhat but may also increase the risk of cancer.[7]

Such serious diseases can occur when free radicals break strands of proteins, creating tissue damage. "This damage prevents the cell from properly taking in nutrients and from properly removing waste products [and in turn] . . . free radical activity inside the cell can alter the replication of the DNA and thereby initiate cancerous changes."[8]

Considering the numerous ways that arthritic conditions are aggravated when we unknowingly consume the wrong foods, I can't help but think of one of Dr. Raymond Peat's explanations of polyunsaturated oils. He writes that they "weaken the immune system's function in ways that are similar to the damage caused by radiation, hormone imbalance, cancer, aging, or viral infections."[9] This view is further illuminated when we look at the numerous studies reporting that unsaturated oils can cause a number of serious diseases.[10] These diseases include immune deficiency,[11] thyroid dysfunction,[12] diabetes, obesity, tumors,[13] heart disease,[14] and white blood cell disorders.[15] (See the list of studies in appendix B.)

On the other hand, when we consume excessive amounts of saturated fats (which predominate in red meats) and combine these with altered unsaturated fats (margarines and shortenings), "our body can't use them properly, and dumps them somewhere. In rheumatism, that place is the muscles and joints."[16] This metabolic instability can also occur when we consume synthetic fat products, such as olestra, which now appear in many processed foods. These chemicals are even more hazardous to our health because they are made up of chemical isolates that are incomplete, unwholesome forms of food. Overuse of these products often leads to disorders, serious allergies, and eventually the malabsorption of nutrients. In *Fats that Heal, Fats that Kill*, Udo Erasmus tells us that "allergic reactions play an important part in *most* arthritic and 'rheumatic' complaints."[17]

## ESSENTIAL FATS FROM PLANT SOURCES

Despite fat-free foods, people are getting heavier and unhealthier. There are several factors that contribute to this. First of all, fat-free foods do not provide satiety and we end up consuming more food, and more calories, in order to get that sense of fullness. Second, fat-free products generally contain more sugar than normal, stimulating the release of insulin, which in turn lowers blood sugar levels. This creates a need to consume more sugar to stabilize blood sugar levels, perpetuating a continuous cycle of eating.

A friend of mine who was trying to lose weight and reduce her cholesterol related this anecdote. As many people do, she began purchasing products with *fat free* and *no cholesterol* on their labels. Unfortunately, terms such as these don't mean the products are highly nutritional or that they are sound food choices. Product advertisers use these labels liberally to increase sales of their product.

My friend wondered why she wasn't losing weight and why she was feeling fatigued. After doing some self-education, she learned how important unrefined and natural fats are in the diet. The next time she went grocery shopping, she looked at the fat-free products and noticed that whenever *fat* had been taken off the product's label, some form of *sugar* had been added.[18] No wonder she was feeling so poorly. She was lacking important nutrients in her diet, nutrients vital to life, health, and energy. She decided to stay away from these products and include foods containing the most beneficial fats, such as extra-virgin olive oil, coconut oil, avocados, walnuts, almonds, and pumpkin seeds. She slowly began feeling more energetic and started losing weight, and her overall health greatly improved.

Dr. Peat has thoroughly reviewed the extensive research concerning fats in the human diet. He points to the harmful effects of too much unsaturated oil, especially the polyunsaturated kind, on all the bodily systems, including oxidative or free radical damage and hormonal imbalance. He alerts us that unsaturated fats cause inflammatory problems, weight gain, and aging.[19]

There is good news, though. Dallas Clouatre, Ph.D., provides data showing the protective role of vitamin C and E supplementation as antioxidants in opposing free radical damage.[20] He emphasizes the need for sticking to fatty acids from plant sources. Dr. Clouatre also suggests substituting fresh raw pumpkin seeds and walnuts for oils and supplementing them with vitamin E for protection against free radicals.[21] The avocado is another source of an important fatty acid that's needed by the body. It contains vitamins E, C, and B, and high levels of potassium, magnesium, zinc, and copper.[22] It is interesting to note that some of the best sources of fats are found in vegetables.[23] Quality fats, high fiber, and whole grains such as barley have never been identified as contributing to any disease.[24]

## AVOID HYDROGENATED FATS

The denatured fats in fried foods, crackers, peanut butter, margarine, most vegetable oils, and many other foods are created by the manufacturer to make a stable shortening. This process, called hydrogenation, enables unsaturated bonds to become saturated with hydrogen when the fats are subjected to a fairly high temperature.[25] This gives the products a longer shelf life, which, of course, makes them more marketable. Author Eustace Mullins explains that "hydrogenated oils in margarine used for cooking break down into dangerous toxins when heated, although butter can be heated for long periods of time without forming toxins."[26] The body cannot tolerate the molecular changes of hydrogenated foods. The creation of trans fatty acids impairs the immune system response by interfering with T cells—the fighters against allergies, infection, cancer, and inflammatory joint disease.[27]

A study that followed 832 men for twenty-one years found that the men, simply by using margarine instead of butter, doubled their risk of allergies and heart disorders, compared with expected results. Other studies by Dr. Peat found that using medications to lower cholesterol while continuing to consume commonly used unsaturated oils led to many forms of serious autoimmune and other diseases.[28] To pursue this research further, refer to appendix B.

Research shows that in addition to adding dyes and preservatives, the manufacturing of margarine creates a synthetic, thus toxic, type of fat that has been linked to joint disease (such as arthritis), heart disease, and other serious diseases.[29] Medical literature explains the mechanism by which "fat toxicity" or other harmful ingredients contribute to some forms of arthritis. For instance, D. A. Lopez, M.D., et al. explain that the body's defense "always involves inflammation and other changes that mislead the immune system." There's much disorder throughout the body, and "chronic rheumatoid arthritis or lupus erythematosus, can themselves extend to the entire vascular system and bring about inflammation."[30]

The deodorizers, solvents, and bleaching compounds used to process these oils contribute to additional trans fatty acids, promoting free radicals. Of course, all fats and oils, whether processed or unrefined, alter when exposed to heat, light, and oxygen. These cause changes that can destroy or block our ability to utilize the essential fatty acids and tocopherols, such as vitamin E.[31] Additionally, they cause fats and oils to become rancid, leading to even more cell-damaging free radical formation—the same factor that has been implicated in arthritis.[32]

The dramatic differences between organic processing and refinement are shown in the diagram that follows. Both methods start with a mechanical cleaning and hulling step (in this case, cleaning and hulling of seeds). For the organic process there is just one other step: The clean seeds are sent through a "cold pressing" system. That produces fresh organic oil, which is bottled in opaque bottles with all nutrients intact. That's it.

For refined oils, the clean seeds are first sent through a crushing

# HOW OILS ARE MANUFACTURED

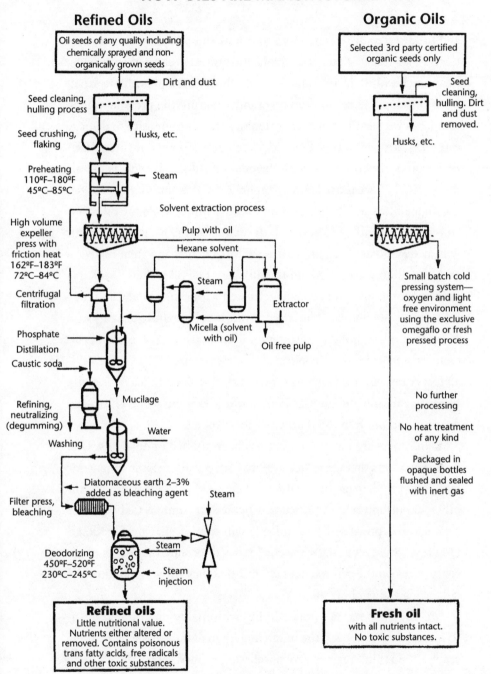

## Refined Oils

Oil seeds of any quality including chemically sprayed and non-organically grown seeds

Dirt and dust

Seed cleaning, hulling process

Husks, etc.

Seed crushing, flaking

Preheating
110ºF–180ºF
45ºC–85ºC

Steam

Solvent extraction process

High volume expeller press with friction heat
162ºF–183ºF
72ºC–84ºC

Pulp with oil

Hexane solvent

Centrifugal filtration

Steam

Micella (solvent with oil)

Extractor

Oil free pulp

Phosphate

Distillation

Caustic soda

Refining, neutralizing (degumming)

Mucilage

Washing

Water

Diatomaceous earth 2–3% added as bleaching agent

Steam

Filter press, bleaching

Deodorizing
450ºF–520ºF
230ºC–245ºC

Steam

Steam injection

### Refined oils
Little nutritional value. Nutrients either altered or removed. Contains poisonous trans fatty acids, free radicals and other toxic substances.

## Organic Oils

Selected 3rd party certified organic seeds only

Seed cleaning, hulling. Dirt and dust removed.

Husks, etc.

Small batch cold pressing system—oxygen and light free environment using the exclusive omegaflo or fresh pressed process

No further processing

No heat treatment of any kind

Packaged in opaque bottles flushed and sealed with inert gas

### Fresh oil
with all nutrients intact. No toxic substances.

*John Finnegan*, The Facts About Fats: A Consumer Guide to Good Oils. *Celestial Arts, Berkeley, California, 1993.*

and flaking step, where exposure to the air can begin to promote rancidity. The "meal" that results from this step is preheated with steam to as much as 180 degrees and then run through a high-volume expeller with temperatures in the same range. During the pressing stages, temperatures vary, but they are often of sufficient intensity to damage essential fatty acids, or EFAs.[33] (Udo Erasmus points out that "EFA deficiencies are correlated with degenerative diseases such as . . . arthritis [and] . . . weakened immune functions.")[34] Some of the oil passes through a filter and then moves on to the distiller, while the oil that is still combined with pulp heads for the extractor. Oil from the extractor is heated with steam again, treated with solvents, and then mixed in with the filtered oil already in the distiller. The oil is then distilled (a process that employs phosphates), treated with caustic soda, and then refined and degummed. The latter step alone eliminates nutrients such as lecithin, phospholipids, protein, polysaccharides, chlorophyll, calcium, magnesium, iron, copper, and any surviving fiber.[35] The oil is almost ready. All that remains is to bleach it with diatomaceous earth, filter it again, deodorize it at temperatures ranging from 450 to 520 degrees, and put it in the bottle. Quite a process.

Consumers are buying oil that has been robbed of nutrients. Udo Erasmus claims that these "unsaturated fatty acids become mutagenic [and] . . . can damage our genes (and those of our offspring)."[36] Another important factor is discussed by author Simone Gabbay, who explains that processed fats and oils will inhibit enzyme function.[37] However, these altered, "synthetic" fats will occupy the spaces of receptor sites on the cell wall and effectively block the action of healthy fatty acids and cholesterol.

Dr. Clouatre warns us that "frying with highly unsaturated oils is so unhealthful that even the much maligned animal fats may be preferable."[38] So think again before purchasing refined vegetable oils, such as margarine rather than butter. Read labels to avoid products containing hydrogenated oils—they are everywhere! When you see the word *hydrogenated*, think of the trans fatty acids created in the hydrogenation process and consider the toll they take on your body.

In addition to the link between trans fatty acid consumption and joint disease associated with arthritis, Dr. Julian Whitaker alerts us to another definite link between trans fatty acids and breast and prostate cancer.[39] Some studies show its relationship to heart disease.[40] In 1950 it was discovered that unsaturated fats suppress the metabolic rate, apparently creating hypothyroidism.[41]

Matthew Gillman, an epidemiologist at Harvard Medical School, has also found research in this area quite disturbing because these trans fatty acids are in all processed foods that contain hydrogenated or partially hydrogenated vegetable oils—including potato chips, cookies, crackers, artificial creamers, mayonnaise, processed salad dressing, most commercially made peanut butter, and most fried foods.[42] According to author and medical reporter Jane Heimlich, the popcorn you buy at the movies or at ballparks is almost always prepared with this partially hydrogenated vegetable oil. Such widespread use of these oils continues to pose an increased health risk for the general population.

Nevertheless, "because the oil industry has powerful lobbies in government, hydrogenation is allowed to continue to supply unnatural fat products to our foods."[43] Dr. Walter Willte at Harvard's School of Public Health informs us that approximately thirty thousand deaths each year may be directly linked to the consumption of these unnatural fats.[44]

The action of a natural or whole food on our body is always more nourishing prior to being altered by high heat, hydrogenation, bleaching, pasteurizing, and other chemicals. These changes alter the nutritive value of food such as those products containing powdered eggs and powdered milk. Physical problems begin to arise when we are regularly ingesting foods that not only are oxidized by industrial processing, but are further oxidized when they are cooked at high temperatures in the presence of light and oxygen.[45]

Don't be misled by the advertising on product labels. It is designed to sell the product, not to help your understanding of good health. Making educated choices about the food you purchase and consume is imperative if you wish to protect yourself from the many forms of degenerative disease now prevalent in our society.

## CHOICES ARE AVAILABLE

With all the research about processed unsaturated fats and their role in many of today's major health disorders, we might well ask, What are the alternatives that will reverse the damage caused by trans fatty acids and free radicals? Dr. Peat finds overwhelming evidence of the destructiveness of an excess of unsaturated oils in the diet and supports the case for saturated fats and, in particular, coconut oil. In fact, we are now discovering that tropical oils such as unrefined coconut oil are healthier than oils from plants grown in colder climates. "This is because tropical plants live at a temperature that is close to our natural body temperature. Tropical oils are stable at high temperatures."[46]

Dr. Peat maintains that when we eat tropical oils, they don't get rancid in our tissues as the cold-climate seed oils, such as corn oil, safflower oil and soy oil, do.[47] Unrefined coconut oil, when added regularly to a balanced diet, lowers cholesterol and actually functions as an antioxidant.[48] William Campbell Douglass, M.D., reports that when this saturated fat is kept at room temperature (even as long as one year) and then tested for rancidity, none is evident.[49] It is even speculated that coconut oil "acts as an antihistamine, an anti-diabetic, [and] an anti-cancer agent."[50]

Coconut oil is the least fattening of all the oils, according to Dr. Peat. He learned that, back in the 1940s, farmers experimented with oils to try to use it to fatten their animals. They used the unrefined (cheapest) coconut oil, but when it was added to the animal feed, the pigs became lean.[51] Not only is it easily metabolized as an energy fuel, but through its action on the thyroid it can increase the general metabolism and bring about the loss of undesirable weight.[52] And when thyroid function is normal, cholesterol levels tend to be normal because cholesterol is being properly converted into hormones and bile salts.

A positive step in reducing our risk of degenerative diseases, including arthritis, is to increase the amount of beneficial saturated fats such as coconut oil in our diet and reduce the unsaturated oils. To clear up any misunderstandings regarding saturated and unsaturated oils, Dr. Peat explains the situation to his reader: "When an oil is saturated, that means that the molecule has all the hydrogen atoms it can hold." Unsaturated oil has some hydrogen atoms missing, and "this opens the structure of the molecule in a way that makes it susceptible to attack by free radicals."[53] All this contributes to aging of the cells. Furthermore, the more unsaturated the fat (polyunsaturated), the greater the exposure to oxidation-creating chain reactions of free radicals.[54] The result is an inflammatory process throughout the body, which too often leads to arthritis, cancer, or autoimmune diseases.

Dr. Peat recommends using unrefined coconut oil or extra-virgin olive oil for their protection against heart disease and other degenerative diseases.[55] The so-called omega-9 (monounsaturated) fatty acids, found in extra-virgin olive oil, also appear to have good properties.

*Extra-virgin olive oil*, derived from the first cold pressing of olives, is safer and more therapeutic than unsaturated vegetable oils for many reasons. First of all, its fatty acid content (80 percent monounsaturated, 12 percent saturated, and 8 percent polyunsaturated) stimulates metabolism and aids digestion. Monounsaturated fatty acids help to lower LDL cholesterol levels and increase HDL levels. In addition, it is made differently from most other vegetable oils (which have to be treated first because the seeds containing toxins are not fit for us to eat) in that the olive itself is ground up and pressed, after which the water is separated from the oil. The untreated extra-virgin olive oil contains the powerful antioxidants vitamin A and vitamin E.[56] Extra-virgin olive oil should not be confused with oil labeled either *virgin olive oil*, which is not from the first pressing and is more acidic, or *100% pure olive oil*, which has been refined in order to neutralize the acidity. Also, when you see the word *light*, it doesn't mean the oil contains less fat. *Light* or *pure* olive oil lacks the distinctive color, taste, and nutrients of extra-virgin olive oil because it no longer retains the oil's original properties.[57]

Olive oil's reputation for improving health comes from the fact that in its unrefined form it contains "phytosterols, chlorophyll, magnesium, vitamin E, carotene," and so much more. This oil contains mainly monounsaturated fatty acids and aids in membrane development—critical to the organs within our body. " 'Extra virgin' means highest quality, and strict guidelines are followed in determining whether an olive oil may be called 'extra virgin.'" We also learn from Udo Erasmus that patients with artery disease who were on low-fat diets switched "from corn oil (refined) to virgin olive oil (unrefined) for six months," resulting in normal cholesterol levels.[58]

This time-tested oil was also found to aid in eliminating toxins from the liver, improve digestion of fats, and even "reduce the production of cholesterol gallstones."[59] Barbara Joseph, M.D., a survivor of breast cancer, tells us that Mediterranean countries customarily use fresh olive or flax oil. "Those populations that consume high levels of olive oil have relatively low breast cancer rates." An extremely important point here is that they use *unheated* fresh olive oil, which is essential in order to preserve the valuable effects.[60]

Some research confirms that alpha-linoleic acid in flaxseed, an omega-3 fatty acid, decreases many inflammatory conditions.[61] These conditions include arthritis, pancreatitis, and tendinitis.[62] Flaxseed is also an excellent source of natural fiber. However, flax oil can rapidly become rancid, posing a real health concern. The best way I have found to buy and consume flaxseed, without being concerned about its rancidity, is to obtain a bag of whole flaxseed and then pulverize the seeds in a coffee grinder. Sprinkle this fresh powder immediately on foods such as salads, cereals, drinks, and so forth. Store in the freezer what you don't use. Consuming this concentrated omega-3, along with its fiber, both of which are lacking in most diets, provides powerful medicinal health benefits. Other safer fats and oils include animal-based fats such as butter and the fat from lamb (if from organic sources).[63]

Next, be sure to include potent antioxidants in your diet, such as flavonoids and vitamins C, E, and A. Some flavonoids that are obtained from plants such as *Ginkgo biloba*, milk thistle, and echinacea have brought beneficial changes to those suffering from inflammatory stress. Some spices and herbs (turmeric, rosemary, garlic, and nutmeg) have even been identified as controlling certain oxidative inflammatory stress disorders.[64]

Other valuable supplements are coenzyme Q10, or Q-gel (which has been found to be three times more bioavailable);[65] minerals such as zinc, selenium,[66] and magnesium; and the enzyme superoxide dismutase[67]—all of which are not found in most Americans' diets. They will provide vital protection from the degenerative process that ultimately leads to arthritis.

Speaking of the fats our body needs, it's interesting to note that butter contains vitamins A, D, and E, selenium, iodine, and cholesterol. These antioxidants not only protect against disease, but are also required for strong bones and teeth.[68] They also assist in the proper absorption of calcium.[69]

A Dutch researcher discovered an antistiffness nutrient in butter.[70] Further documentation reveals that this vital substance found in unpasteurized butter can actually protect against joint calcification, degenerative arthritis, hardening of the arteries, and cataracts. If using butter products concerns you, consider that another study reported that "calves fed . . . skim milk develop joint stiffness . . . . Their symptoms are reversed when raw butterfat is added to the diet."[71] Perhaps the national craze for avoiding fat is misguided.

Speaking of butter, I have found ghee, a golden oil with a buttery taste, to be quite spreadable at room temperature. Ghee is actually clarified butter, but it is lactose free because the milk-fat solids and water are removed. It also has a long shelf life and does not become rancid. Ghee has been used for thousands of years in India not only for cooking (it doesn't smoke or burn in the process), but also for medicinal purposes. Health reporter Cheryl Player writes that "According to Rudolph Ballentine, M.D., ghee contains an ideal, balanced ratio of fatty acids and contains no transfatty acids which are associated with heart disease." She explains that ghee contains a fatty acid called butyric acid, which combats a variety of serious diseases. She continues, "Ghee acts as a vital carrier of medicinals to the tissues of the body [and] has long been used as a base for herbal remedies. In this way, the medicine penetrates deep into tissue layers enhancing absorption."[72]

## FISH OILS AND ARTHRITIS

A study published in *The New England Journal of Medicine* documents that fish oils possess anti-inflammatory agents that are beneficial to patients suffering from rheumatoid arthritis.[73] Both Dr. Julian Whitaker and Dr. Jason Theodosakis confirm that these oils, high in omega-3 fatty acids, reduce both the inflammation and the related pain often manifested with arthritis.[74] In one study, when patients consumed fish on a daily basis they had less swelling, joint discomfort, and fatigue.[75]

Clinical trials have been published on the therapeutic effect of eicosapentaenoic acid and docosahexaenoic acid from fish oils, and how these fatty acids can alleviate inflammatory problems such as rheumatoid arthritis, psoriasis, and bowel disease.[76] These oils seem to function so well in the human body because they are also constituents of our own cells—the brain, nerve synapses, retina, and other "biochemically active tissues in our body."[77]

Several sources that fish oil is good for cardiovascular disease, but one recently published states that "fish and fish oil have swum beyond lipids and cardiovascular health. Recent studies also indicate that they have beneficial effects on arthritis, breast cancer, Crohn's disease, and asthma."[78]

Some believe that the regular intake of the omega-3 fats contained in fish is the reason Inuits don't have cholesterol problems. Their consumption of marine fat "creates a cellular situation that overpowers other fat's ability to trigger heart and other chronic diseases." This diet also regulates prostaglandin activity by blocking certain enzymes that induce inflammation. This produces an effect similar to that produced by aspirin and other anti-inflammatory drugs. It regulates the underlying metabolic mechanisms that set off pain associated with inflammation.[79]

Some of the cold-water fish that are particularly high in omega-3 fatty acids, and have been found to combat various forms of arthritis, are salmon, sardines, mackerel, trout, and tuna.[80] Their oils are not only useful in combating arthritis,[81] but are rich in protein and iodine, and they are beneficial for thyroid function. They also increase antibacterial factors in the blood.[82] Keep in mind, however, that not all fish oils contain these health-enhancing fatty acids.[83]

Jane Heimlich tells us about Dale Alexander, who is a strong advocate of using fresh "cod liver oil [as] a 'key weapon' in controlling arthritis." It has been used for this purpose for over two hundred years.[84] Alexander says, "Arthritis is a disease of dryness."[85] Because cod-liver oil may increase one's requirement for vitamin E, a good alternative is halibut-liver oil capsules.[86] We are learning that essential fatty acids "are necessary to produce secretions that lubricate our joints. They are also required to build and deposit bone material, and to transport minerals."[87] While some oils and fats, in moderation, protect our cells, chemically altered fats hold cholesterol in the blood. This cholesterol accumulation weakens the integrity of our cells, contributing to a variety of degenerative diseases. Is it any wonder that we eventually feel bad after eating the standard American diet?

## EMU OIL

Emu oil has proven beneficial for arthritis, and I believe it's an oil we'll be hearing more about in the near future as word gets around. This oil has been used as a therapeutic agent for thousands of years by the aboriginal tribes of Australia. It is derived from the layer of fat found on the back of the emu. It was mainly used for muscular and joint pain. A small clinical study of twenty people found definite anti-inflammatory properties in emu oil and concluded that it was beneficial for arthritis patients.[88]

Research has not revealed any adverse side effects from the consumption of bacteria-free emu oil.[89] In fact, U.S. patent documentation found that emu oil improved lipid profiles by decreasing total cholesterol, triglycerides, and low-density lipoproteins (LDLs) and increasing high-density lipoproteins (HDLs) when used on a regular basis. It also exhibits a longer shelf life than most other oils because it has all the properties of a long-chain fatty acid despite being a short-chain fatty acid.[90]

Emu oil may be used topically and orally for inflammation resulting in musculoskeletal or dermatological conditions from environmental or systemic causes.[91] Since it can be used topically, it's beneficial not only for arthritic conditions, but also for skin disorders such as eczema, burns, and lesions.[92]

Other reports concluded that although emu oil fights anti-inflammatory conditions close to the surface of the skin, it "must be mixed with a 'carrier,' such as alcohol or essential plant oils, which will transport it through the skin to inflamed tissues."[93] Another opinion comes from Dr. William Code of British Columbia who specializes in pain control. He was impressed with how well emu oil was absorbed into the skin. He says he personally uses it for muscle and joint aches, abrasions, and burns.[94]

The editor of *Emu Today and Tomorrow* also writes about yet another medical practitioner who began serious investigation into this oil when his patients spoke of its benefits. As a physician in family practice, Dr. Howard Hagglund discovered that "emu oil keeps the joint warm and doesn't overheat it." He also found the oil to be natural, safe, penetrating, and therapeutic for sports injuries, aching feet, and aching muscles.[95]

## FRIEND OR FOE IN CHOLESTEROL?

Cholesterol plays a critical role in the body's healing process. It is a crystalline, fat-soluble steroid alcohol. It's found in greatest concentration in animal foods such as meat, particularly liver and other organ meats, eggs, shellfish, and full-fat dairy products.[96] In *Health Freedom News* we read, "Cholesterol is an integral part of the cell structure. . . . Animal cells owe their shape and firmness to cholesterol. . . . Cholesterol is nature's healing substance."[97]

John Finnegan, N.D., states that "over eight percent of our brain's solid matter is made of cholesterol." We are learning that it's used for a variety of purposes, such as the formation of the myelin sheath, the protective coating that surrounds our nerves. Dr. Finnegan continues, "Our hormones, skin, and even the membranes of our cells use cholesterol as an essential building block in their basic production and structure."[98] If we experience trauma and injury, such as sprains, tears, or ruptures, the body produces a surplus of cholesterol so that healing can take place.[99]

Cholesterol is a fatty substance that can be synthesized in the body from saturated fats, as well as from carbohydrates and protein. We obtain some cholesterol from our food, but it is also produced within the body.[100] And while the danger of high cholesterol levels is well publicized, the reverse can also be a problem. It has been discovered, for instance, that low serum cholesterol levels can be linked with digestive tract disease, nervous disorders, and cerebral hemorrhages.[101] William Regelson, M.D., and Carol Colman report, "People with very low cholesterol levels are more likely to develop cancer or to suffer from mental illness."[102]

Discussing the danger of high cholesterol has become commonplace in health reporting, and it is definitely a risk factor for heart attack. But we need to look a little further. There are two major components to your cholesterol count: LDL, which is often considered the "bad" cholesterol, and HDL, which is referred to as the "good" one. While an extremely high level of total cholesterol can be dangerous in itself, it is more commonly the HDL-LDL ratio that is critical. In fact, higher levels of HDLs are essential for normal function. HDLs act as an antioxidant in the body and also remove excess cholesterol from the blood.[103] HDLs are also required for the production of vitamin D, which allows not only calcium absorption, but also bile production, which is necessary for the breakdown of fats from our diet.

Our body has a feedback mechanism that increases or reduces the amount of cholesterol we produce, *provided we don't overconsume starches, sugars, and trans fat.*[104] This is demonstrated by the fact that the body only uses about 20 to 40 percent of the cholesterol supplied by the food we eat.[105] In other words, if blood cholesterol rises above a certain level, the excess is converted into bile and excreted in the stool.[106]

High cholesterol can be controlled by natural means—by increasing fiber, antioxidants, and exercise, along with reducing hydrogenated oils and refined sugar. Drugs that lower cholesterol levels can cause serious side effects such as muscle pain, intestinal disorders, headaches, insomnia, liver damage, and even cancer.[107]

High cholesterol (above 250) may be a risk factor for heart disease, but it's not the only one. There are people who have high LDL-HDL cholesterol levels and still live to a ripe old age without any heart disease whatsoever, just as there are those with low cholesterol ratios who suddenly die of a heart attack before they even reach age forty.[108] Let's look beyond the total cholesterol number for the real picture.

Because people have been misinformed about cholesterol they have avoided many wholesome foods that can produce the right balance of cholesterol in the body. This in turn has caused immune deficiency diseases and may even have cost lives.[109] Sometimes it's not the food we're eating, hereditary influences, lack of exercise, or any of the other usual suspects, but rather a malfunctioning liver that's the cause of high cholesterol. The liver is responsibile for cleansing the bloodstream of cholesterol. If the liver is malfunctioning, LDL cholesterol can be forced to recirculate, causing a high-cholesterol profile.

To the extent that a cholesterol imbalance is due to a sluggish liver, those concerned about their cholesterol might want to try Dr. Richard Schulze's liver-gallbladder flush. This tonic consists of 8 oz fresh citrus juice, 8 oz distilled water, one to five cloves of garlic (add one more each day), one to five tablespoons of organic extra-virgin olive oil, and an inch-long piece of fresh gingerroot, mixed together in the blender. It is taken for five consecutive mornings, and consumed in less than five minutes, followed by two cups of a detoxifying tea fifteen minutes later. Dr. Schulze makes the tea out of Oregon grape rootbark, gentian root, wormwood leaves, and dandelion root.[110]

Sometimes when we neglect to routinely detoxify our body, the body will do it for us: It will detoxify itself through a fever. A fever is a sign that the body is slowly killing the microorganisms that create disease. An elevated body temperature actually destroys bacteria. Fever and sweating increase the speed with which toxins are expelled. A fever is nature's way of helping the body rid itself of toxins. Although the process is uncomfortable, it provides a useful service by unlocking the deep roots of the disease.

## FRIENDLY FOODS INDEED

We are typically told to avoid specific foods in order to keep cholesterol levels low. Sometimes, however, we may be avoiding the wrong foods. An example of this is found in a study from Denmark concerning the role of eggs in the diet. Dr. Earl Mindell provides us with a startling research finding: "When 21 healthy adults ranging in ages from 23 to 52 years old were given two boiled (not fried) eggs every day plus their ordinary diet, their good blood cholesterol [HDL] went up 10 percent while their total blood cholesterol only went up 4 percent after six weeks."[111] Most doctors are now beginning to conclude that moderate egg consumption may be beneficial, especially when compared with disorders associated with low-fat, no-cholesterol diets, which reduce both HDL and LDL cholesterol.

Judy McFarland, author of *Aging Without Growing Old*, reminds us that eggs, "the most perfect food that God put upon this earth, the food for the embryo, the food associated with new life, [have] taken the brunt of the cholesterol scare."[112] Saturated fats, in fact, have been known to increase serum cholesterol levels more significantly than eggs.[113]

Incidentally, Dr. Peat mentions in his book *Nutrition for Women* that including eggs and liver in the diet will promote the formation of progesterone, because cholesterol acts as a precursor to this molecule.[114] How many of us have considered that cholesterol is essential to the production of our hormones? How many of us realize that pregnenolone, the precursor to all our hormones, is made in our body directly from cholesterol?[115] For more details on this key subject of the relationship between cholesterol and pregnenolone, refer to chapter 6.

## "FAT FREE": PROMOTION AND PROPAGANDA

So why is cholesterol getting such a bad rap when it performs so many wonderful functions in keeping us healthy? The truth is that what's done to fats and oils is the real culprit. The molecular changes, additives, artificial coloring, and preservatives in processed products are the enemy, not cholesterol. Dr. Finnegan warns: "Diets have become seriously deficient in key minerals, vitamins, fiber, amino acids, and often complex carbohydrates. Yet only now is it becoming generally understood that modern processing methods of fats and oils have created even more serious damage from poisonous rancid oils and trans-fatty acids, as well as deficiencies of Omega-3 and Omega-6 fatty acids and certain prostaglandins. . . . The body is made from and requires cholesterol and the Omega-3 and Omega-6 fatty acids."[116]

The omega-6 fatty acids, however, that are obtained from pork, chicken, and beef can generate inflammatory prostaglandins, says Patricia Clarke, M.D. And these hormonelike substances can intensify inflammation in the joints. On the other hand, vegetable and omega-3 fat consumption will help nourish cartilage and joint health.[117] But, unfortunately, consuming processed foods rich in refined fat and sugar is the more prevailing lifestyle in America, and it is one of the major factors in arthritic problems in people of all ages. It would be helpful to consumers to be told the truth about foods.

## THE SEARCH BRINGS GOOD RESULTS

As we proceed through life, illness often serves to alert us to the fact that medicine is often found in nature and there is seldom a need to be dependent on synthetic drugs. Through education we can build up the confidence we need to make independent and wise decisions. We no longer need to be tempted by the endless choices of commercial products extravagantly packaged, yet devoid of life. We can easily be influenced by these external persuasions, but with the power of education, we can finally experience the excitement of making our own choices. And this freedom to choose what is in tune with the body's needs is a gift of life.

# Nerve Interference and Degenerative Arthritis (Joint Care through Chiropractic)

*Life force may be the least*
*understood force on this earth.*

**Norman Cousins**

The extraordinary accomplishments of the medical profession are well known. Myriad feats—reconstructive surgery, skin and bone grafting, organ and joint transplants—seem like modern miracles, and M.D.'s seem like the miracle workers. They heroically rescue victims of heart attacks, wounds to vital organs, life-threatening tumors, obstructions, gangrenous limbs, severed tendons or arteries, broken bones, brain hemorrhages. This country owes a great debt to the medical profession, and most of its citizens, rightly, have the highest regard for medical doctors.

However, when it comes to detecting nutritional starvation, natural hormone deficiency, and nerve interference, the orthodox establishment has much to learn. The entire area of natural healing has been left out of the curriculum offered to most medical students.

Fortunately more and more medical doctors are independently moving beyond the prevailing orthodox medical practice in order to pursue greater truth for the benefit of humanity.

Let's take a look at two of the time-honored therapies that have been shown to help prevent disease by increasing the response of the immune system: cleansing (detoxifying), and restoring structural and nutritional homeostasis. In acute stages of illness, there is a need to purge toxicity from the body in order to maintain structural balance and healthy joints. This often involves multiple methods that complement one another. These varied and gentle ways of healing don't need a prescription.

There are a number of such options to choose from: herbalism (including ayurvedic or Chinese medicine), homeopathy, acupuncture, Shiatsu, naturopathy, aromatherapy, chelation, hyperthermia, osteopathy, and so on—and of course the largest licensed natural health care profession in the United States, chiropractic. Andrew Taylor Still, the father of osteopathy, states the goal of that profession best: "A perfectly adjusted body which will produce pure blood and plenty of it, deliver it on time and in quantity sufficient to supply all demands in the economy of life."[1]

Chiropractic care enhances nerve flow. The nervous system is the major regulator for all hormonal performances. This is because the spinal nerves and the endocrine system are critically interconnected.[2] The nervous system controls the immune system in its effort to fight systemic diseases such as arthritis.[3] Conditions of spinal misalignments and subsequent nerve interference should always be addressed, because they influence each mental and physical function.[4]

A doctor of chiropractic is professionally trained to understand why poor diet, hormone imbalances, and, most particularly, nerve interference may contribute to disease. A well-trained chiropractor can detect and correct nerve impingement caused by spinal misalignments. Spinal correction eventually enables the body to improve regulation of the immune, secretory, excretory, and motor systems. According to Tedd Koren, D.C., "Recent research has shown that chiropractic care can reverse some of the effects of osteoarthritis—something which had been previously considered impossible."[5]

Signs of arthritis do not appear suddenly; they develop over time. We learn from *The Primer on the Rheumatic Diseases* that the disease may occur at any time although the risk of developing it increases with age.[6] In osteoarthritis, degenerative processes begin in the joint cartilage or disc and can spread to the nearby bone. These changes often lead to the formation of painful bone spurs.[7] Gradually, the disease is felt as pain in various joints and in the related soft tissue. Pain commonly occurs in places like the knuckles of the hand and the knee, or in a vertebra that may have misaligned from a sprain or strain caused by an earlier fall or accident.

If one waits too long to have an osteoarthritic spine adjusted back into alignment, the discs between the two vertebrae will begin to decrease in height, bringing these two bones closer together. As this continues, lipping, spurring, or even disc herniations may develop as the body attempts to reinforce and protect the area.[8] Ultimately, bony fusion between vertebrae may result.

I personally found that accurate and precise adjustments enhance communication between the central nervous system and every cell in the body.[9] A hundred years ago, Thomas Edison echoed a similar theme when he predicted, "The doctor of the future will give no medicine, but will interest his patients in the care of the human frame, in diet, and in the cause and prevention of disease."[10] The future is now here for those in tune with this natural alternative. In fact, chiropractic has become "the fastest growing health care profession in the world."[11] It has given millions of patients the freedom to live an active life and has provided hope to countless others in critical need.[12]

Stuart M. Berger, M.D., in his book *What Your Doctor* Didn't *Learn in Medical School*, says that there is most likely a complex, interrelated web involving the nervous, endocrine, and immune systems, each acting on its own as well as reacting to the operation of the others.[13] Perhaps a similar, or the same, illness may be named differently depending on which specialist is diagnosing and describing it. There are such a variety of specialties in this area of medicine—immunologists, cardiologists, endocrinologists, gastroenterologists, neurologists, and many more—that it is no wonder similar illnesses may be diagnosed and treated differently, and as separate entities.

But just as methods of healing interact, so do diseases; and virtually all disease represents a complex interaction between outside causative agents (bacteria, viruses, and so forth) and the internal state of the patient's body. Any treatment is much more effective when it addresses all of these factors. If part of the treatment is missing, imbalance and disease may very well prevail. If one of the systems of the body begins to malfunction, it could create illness in a different area.

## THE BODY COMPENSATES TO SURVIVE

One disorder often leads to another, and seemingly unrelated problems may stem from a common cause. For example, Edward McDonagh, D.O., tells us that 1.2 million osteoporotic fractures occur every year in the United States. And whether the women experiencing these fractures are on estrogen therapy seems to have no effect on the rate of incidence. "Other prescribed medications such as anticonvulsants, anticoagulants, cortisone, antacids, diuretics, and many cancer medications contribute to bone loss. In addition, cigarettes and excess of alcohol have been reported to promote osteoporosis." A loss of bone mineral density creates weaker bones[14] and a variety of joint problems including decreased joint space. When all this is combined with poor lifestyle choices such as improper nutrition or lack of exercise, arthritic symptoms such as pain, inflammation, and swelling may occur.

Arthritis is not an isolated disease, and it cannot be treated in isolation from other disorders of the body. The treatment that we choose should take into consideration the body as a whole, not just the particular joints that ache.[15] This is one reason why chiropractic care should be considered, and why painkillers and other short-term solutions do not fix the underlying cause.[16]

When any of the spinal vertebrae are misaligned, there will be interference to the nerve flow that supplies the organs and joints throughout the body. These *subluxations*, as they're called, can cause our organs to function poorly.[17] Back pain or arthritic conditions may originate from a trivial incident, or from whiplash, the birthing process, an old sports injury, an automobile accident, or any trauma of this sort. Every time I hear an ambulance siren, I think, "This could very well be the start of a long journey to future health problems for some-one—emotional as well as physical."

We often fail to associate an ailment with the specific event or trauma that caused it. Pain and mysterious disorders come and go, as the spinal cord tries to compensate for the changes introduced to the body through injury or misuse. The need to be adjusted isn't always immediately apparent at the time because sometimes we don't feel the local pain in our joints or spine. But, on the other hand, we "just don't feel well." If this condition goes untreated for months or years, the inflammatory process and age-related diseases set in.[18]

I was finally forced to listen to my body when my symptoms became too painful to ignore. Experience taught me that quick fixes in the name of healing only traded short-term relief for long-term discomfort.[19] As time went on I also learned to first heed the warning signals by searching alternative ways for addressing the cause (not just the symptoms) of my disorders in order to allow the body to heal itself. Learning to listen to the body will help to avoid back and other joint problems in the future. By removing the nerve interference, *time* will once again do wonders in assisting the body to heal itself.[20]

## MY PERSONAL AWAKENING

I had my share of sports injuries as a skier and tennis player when I was younger, but I didn't suffer from any back pain or arthritis during those very active years. But the painless subluxations were occurring—most likely brought on by a combination of a few hard falls on the Alpine ski slopes and the difficult labor and delivery of my child. Looking back, I now understand that over time these and other normal life experiences triggered further misalignments, bringing on more serious health problems.

As anyone who has been there knows, the birthing process alone can be very traumatic to both the mother and child.[21] Two months following the birth of my son, the left side of my body became paralyzed from a blood clot that originated somewhere in my body and finally lodged in my brain. My neurosurgeon and other doctors were completely puzzled and said, "But she's only thirty-five—too young for a stroke!" Way back then there was no Dr. John Lee or Dr. Katharina Dalton at hand to enlighten my specialist about why new mothers may suffer from either postpartum depression or, as in my case, blood clotting in the presence of high estrogen and cortisol levels. Low levels of progesterone can occur after any trauma and result in a hormonal imbalance—especially after giving birth. In chapter 6, we will cover in greater detail how this imbalance can also affect joint and bone health.

I was fortunate. I slowly recovered, and my body was rehabilitated through many sessions of physical therapy and nutritional support. But the intermittent pain in my hip continued to worsen through the years, convincing me that I was destined to be arthritic for the rest of my life. I also began to suffer from menstrual disorders and was told a hysterectomy would be necessary. Second and third opinions supported the finding. I was simultaneously suffering from what some doctors called "arthritic" back and leg pain. When I told my orthopedist that I'd heard of a good chiropractor and would like to try this type of care before committing to surgery, he strongly advised me against it. He suggested instead that I go to the pain clinic and learn how to "live with my pain."

Fortunately, I did not take his advice and instead, in desperation, made an appointment with the chiropractor, who specialized in upper cervical health care. To my complete surprise—after nearly twelve years of "living with it"—the severe back and sciatic pain went away. Recently, I found a few of the many studies that explained why.[22] I learned that this technique, involving precise analysis of the atlas (first cervical vertebrae), restored body balance and proper nerve flow so that organs, limbs, and tissues were able to function normally again. The profession that I was told could cripple or paralyze me gave me back my health. It was one of the most wonderful experiences of my life. For the first time in years I was able to sleep soundly through the night. But more than that, my "bursitis" and "tendinitis" cleared up, conditions I had been treating with cortisone shots. I was truly amazed when I no longer suffered from chronic gynecological problems. I realize now it was no coincidence that my uterine and cervical disorders occurred simultaneously with my sciatica.[23]

The following drawings illustrate why tension, which can result from accidents, sickness, or stress, can originate from a single bone being out of alignment at the top of the spinal cord. This imbalance can restrict messages that flow from the brain to that part of the body serviced by these nerves and thus create overall musculoskeletal difficulties. When correction is made and the body is once again in balance, pressure is released from the spinal cord and the body is able to heal itself.

Following this experience, I slowly became stronger, both mentally and physically. I resolved to divert all the energy that was creating resentment of my misdiagnosis and mistreatment into positive energy directed at spreading vital information about this gentle, noninvasive care that brought me back to health. I dedicated myself to spreading

## Body Balance

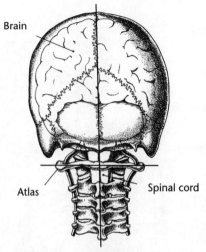

Brain

Atlas

Spinal cord

*A spinal correction balances the bone structure of the head and neck.*
*This relieves the spinal cord distortion and allows the body*
*to return to a state of balance.*

## Body Imbalance

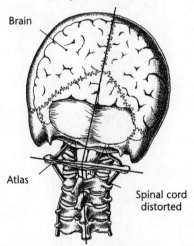

Brain

Atlas

Spinal cord
distorted

*Stress, trauma, or accidents pull the head and neck off balance.*
*This misalignment creates tension on the spinal cord and*
*distorts the nerve supply to the body. This body imbalance can*
*cause pain, suffering, and poor health.*

# Here's What Happens

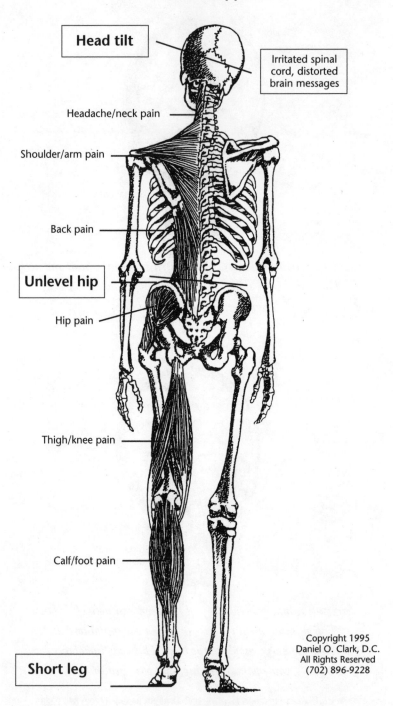

Head tilt

Irritated spinal cord, distorted brain messages

Headache/neck pain

Shoulder/arm pain

Back pain

Unlevel hip

Hip pain

Thigh/knee pain

Calf/foot pain

Short leg

the word about the benefits of chiropractic to help others who suffer from neck, knee, shoulder, or other joint pain.[24] And the fact that the medical establishment's practitioners were universally hostile to these alternatives made me all the more determined to speak out.

This all began as far back as 1943, when some of the more successful chiropractors were sentenced to jail for practicing medicine without a license, though they never prescribed medicine or recommended surgery. This was partly due to the fact that many states did not have licensure for chiropractic. Years of persecution were thrust on these doctors who wished to pursue their profession, knowing that the correct adjustment relieved the relentless and endless suffering of their patients.[25]

The results these doctors produced threatened orthodox medicine. In 1963 the American Medical Association (AMA) began to "overtly and covertly" (words of the Court) eliminate the profession of chiropractic in the United States.[26]

On August 27, 1987, the results of lengthy trials in May and June were revealed in a 101-page document. This opinion found that the AMA and its members participated in a conspiracy against chiropractors in violation of the nation's antitrust laws. Thereafter an opinion dated September 25, 1987 was substituted for the one granted on August 27.[27] In it the United States District Court Judge Susan Getzendanner ordered the AMA, along with 275,000 members, from "restricting, regulating or impeding . . . the freedom of any AMA members or any institution or hospital to make an individual decision as to whether or not that AMA member, institution or hospital shall professionally associate with chiropractors, chiropractic students, or chiropractic institutions."[28] For more information about the antitrust suit go to www.chirobase.org.

The AMA was convicted of conspiracy to control and abolish the chiropractic practice in the United States and was found guilty of impeding fair competition in the health field. The lawsuit was finally settled for the wrongful slander of chiropractic by the AMA.

Actually, much good came from this trial. It finally provided national publicity for one of the valuable paths to good health. People learned from those who testified before the court how chiropractors actually helped. I for one was motivated to report what I had learned. In 1992 my "mission impossible," a book entitled *Today's Health Alternative*, was published. Writing has never been my forte. This miracle was accomplished through sheer determination coupled with the teamwork of wonderful and talented friends who shared the same purpose.

As I explain in *Today's Health Alternative*, the interruption of nerve impulses (which can be caused by stress, or poor posture or sleeping position) can be the underlying cause of a weakened immune system, digestive disorders, and, of course, arthritic conditions.[29] Sooner or later these problems will surface. My personal experience with chiropractic adjustments gave me back my physical health and a greater mental awareness that I had not experienced since my youth. This care helped me to live without drugs and surgery and was an ever present reminder of how the mind, body, and spirit must all work together to create a truly healthy person. The best health bonus was the disappearance of my seasonal flu and colds. They never surfaced again. Even my child's neuromuscular coordination improved; and allergies, asthma, and severe coughing became less severe.[30]

Coincidence? It doesn't appear so. Studies show that there is a cause and effect relationship between chiropractic care and overall health. After many sleepless nights, my anxieties resulting from ill health became a thing of the past. What I once thought was a mystery I now understand differently. It is a *science*![31] Over the years, I learned from personal experience that time does heal when joint misalignments have been corrected throughout the body.[32] But releasing nerve interference in the spine especially aids in joint health and the prevention of disorders down the road that could lead to arthritis. There are many wonderful precise and gentle chiropractic techniques for adjusting even the small bones in the extremities and throughout the body. This was amazing to me, especially since I had been brought up in a medically oriented family who thought chiropractors couldn't help you. Knowing this is the prevailing attitude was one of the driving forces behind my writing this book.

## THE ROOT CAUSE LEFT UNATTENDED

As we noted previously, most allopathic (i.e., Western medicine) doctors help us in a variety of ways, but they have not been trained to detect or correct vertebral subluxations, misalignments of the spine that create pressure on nerves within the central nervous system. This interruption or interference in the nervous system's signals can cause immune and circulatory problems such as vague discomfort throughout the whole body and blood pressure disorders.[33]

With children, subluxations can result in sudden infant death syndrome (SIDS).[34] After all, the birthing process is traumatic to the infant too. If spinal misalignment is not addressed, frequent illnesses or health problems may result. Instead of just saying the baby will outgrow symptoms, health problems should be heeded as a warning. Alternatives should be considered before childhood arthritis or other physical or mental disorders such as learning disabilities and attention span disorders manifest themselves.[35]

The spinal column is the housing unit for the nervous system and we need to focus more attention on misalignments and imbalances. If proper diagnosis and correction were provided in hospitals, our children would experience a much healthier head start. The good news is that today chiropractors are residents in over one hundred fifty of the country's approximately six thousand hospitals, and increasingly hospitals are actively recruiting doctors of chiropractic.[36] The age of chiropractic will come soon, but for now I think it's extremely negligent not to have a good chiropractor in every hospital and pain clinic.

When proper spinal care, which stimulates our body's own

extraordinary resources, becomes more commonplace, dependency on prescription drugs or the use of exploratory surgery, which is now routinely practiced in hospitals, may be drastically reduced. When that time comes, "The winner in all of this, for the first time, will be the patient," says Dr. Louis Sportelli.[37] Both infants and mothers should be checked for neuromusculoskeletal disorders both before and after the birth process. An ounce of such prevention may avoid years of future neurological stress, mental anxieties,[38] age-related disorders, and eventually joint pain and arthritis.[39]

Upper cervical trauma sustained during birth is common in infants. In Germany Dr. G. Gutman examined and adjusted more than a thousand infants with atlas blockage.[40] He states his conclusions in *Manuelle Medizin*: "Blocked nerve impulses at the atlas [top vertebra] cause many clinical features from central motor impairment to lower[ed] resistance to infections—especially ear, nose and throat infections. . . . Chiropractic can often bring about amazingly successful results because the therapy is a causal one."[41] If this nerve transmission disorder is not corrected, who knows how this injury will affect other parts of the body later in life. Sadly, we are even beginning to hear about several types of childhood arthritis. Juvenile rheumatoid arthritis (JRA) has become one of the most common forms of such arthritic conditions and can develop in children under sixteen years of age.[42]

As stated previously, NSAIDs, gold treatments, and aspirin are often given "to reduce the pain and inflammation, and antibiotics if the triggering infection is known."[43] But it would be much better, or wiser, if we were first referred to a chiropractor who specializes in restoring joint function. Toxic drug treatments can cause kidney, liver, or intestinal disorders,[44] as well as destruction to bone and cartilage,[45] encouraging joints to become a battleground for further stress.

More government funds should be allotted to natural and alternative ways of healing instead of being committed entirely to areas such as vaccinations, mammograms, medications, and treatments that don't stimulate the innate power within our bodies for self-healing.[46] As we have seen in the numerous studies cited throughout this book, when we focus on "medicating the disease" rather than "preventing the disease," long-range traumatic side effects can result from toxic residue accumulation in cells and, too often, in the joints themselves.

## JOINT DISEASE WITHIN OUR GRASP

It's time to seek natural alternatives and discover the underlying causes of joint disease. More often than not, our discomforts are associated with nerve interruption, nutritional deficiency, hormonal deficiency, or possibly all three. This is emphasized in an article in *Woman's Day* entitled "What You Should Know About Your Glands." John W. Tintera, M.D., reminds us that for generations science has shown the nervous system to be the lead coordinator of all body functions working intimately with the endocrine system.[47] Leon Chaitow N.D., D.O., further explains that this vital interconnection encompasses a balance between not only the biochemical system but also the structural system (which includes muscles, blood vessels, and organs) and, of course, the emotions and spiritual processes. When all of these are in balance we can achieve homeostasis. However, where a deficiency exists within any of these systems, there is a lack of interplay that can bring on stress and poor health.[48]

And so it is that many people today, dissatisfied with the standard medical treatments, have chosen to disregard recommendations that do not promote natural healing. Some of them have sought relief in a health care that evolved from the principles of Hippocrates. This famed practitioner of drugless healing advised his students to acquire a knowledge of the spine as a prerequisite for the understanding of many diseases!

Despite official resistance by their professional organizations, increasing numbers of medical doctors have joined with their patients in acknowledging that traditional medicine does not have all the answers.

They recognize the higher goal: to make people healthier. The newly initiated are discovering that today's chiropractic methods are varied and diverse; that in addition to the more commonly known techniques, there are now adjustments that employ very light force. For many what was once the last resort has now become their first recourse when not feeling well.[49]

When we are well again, we no longer have to focus on our ailments or be governed by medication. Instead we become more independent and self-motivated in seeking health care choices. In this healthier state of mind, we are better able to  help others to cope with the stresses of life and in turn, to become more involved in our communities and families.

We can most particularly become more active in speaking out on health reform. A good place to start is by lobbying your congresspeople to expand the National Institutes of Health Office of Alternative Medicine and increase public funding for research into alternative medical therapies. Help is also needed to restrain the Food and Drug Administration from blindly maligning cost-effective natural compounds that are proven to help heal arthritis and other diseases. Federal funds should go toward researching the many natural alternatives that are not only well founded scientifically, but also work!

## SEARCHING FOR MORE LOGICAL ANSWERS

Are we going to the wrong doctors because they are the doctors our insurance programs cover? Are we being misdiagnosed because we are going to the wrong specialist? The answers to these questions bring me to why I fell into the misdiagnosis/mistreatment trap, and became a victim of my own ignorance. Desperation drove me to a specialist. The neurologists, such as the one I went to years ago, checked for nerve disorder by means of electromyography testing (EMG). The EMG has been found to have poor sensitivity. It will only tell the doctor the nerve has been damaged; it only tests the motor portion of the nerve root. Many back problems or back pain involve the sensory and afferent portion of the root.[50] My test indicated that there was no problem (except perhaps in my head).

Hip and knee replacements as well as back surgery are now offered to many as the only options to relieve symptoms even though obtaining a second opinion from a specialist in neuromusculoskeletal and biomechanical conditions (an osteopath, chiropractor, physical therapist, and so forth) could actually be a safer and more logical choice. Misalignments are often found to be the cause of not only back pain, but also other diseases.[51]

Unfortunately, this wiser approach of checking for nerve interference is not normally practiced, although more and more medical doctors are recognizing the benefits of more gentle and conservative care. In many cases, surgical treatment is only the beginning of further disorders down the road.

Following surgery, a patient may be given prescription(s) to treat symptoms of pain. It may be, though, that the pain is originating from undetected spinal *nerve interference*. Without attending to this area first, it is no wonder that a patient may not respond to medication and may continue to deteriorate, becoming frail, arthritic, and osteoporotic.[52]

So let's give our spirit a chance to live by thinking twice about blindly accepting whatever orthodox medicine has to offer. Patients continue to speak out on this because experience has shown them that this natural care of relieving nerve pressure works in alleviating many of our disorders. Now the insurance companies and government agencies should acknowledge the public's needs and provide both chiropractic and other natural therapies on an as-needed basis, or better yet, for preventive care.

Why should we spend time seeking natural therapies that will improve our physical health? The answer is summed up in this quotation: "A person should take every care of his body . . . not for the sake of the body, but in order that the soul in a sound body may act . . . rightly, and may have the body as an organ perfectly obedient to it."[53] These inspired words of eighteenth-century scientist, philosopher, and theologian Emanuel Swedenborg influenced my own philosophy of life and strengthened my determination to work ever so much more closely with those who also wish to improve the quality of their lives on all planes—the physical, emotional, and, ultimately, the spiritual.

The right doctor can gently release the healing potential that exists within the human body. It is this innate force that manifests itself on the mind and body in positive and effective ways. With the help of this hidden higher power the body will then heal itself!

# 6
# Hormonal Deficiency Leading to Arthritis

*Eliminating the cause by restoring*
*balance will produce a true cure.*

**Raymond Peat, Ph.D.**

Nutritional and hormonal deficiencies are becoming an increasing health concern in the world today. They are a primary focus in newspaper health columns, health stores, medical doctors' newsletters, articles on alternative treatments in medical journals and books, and, of course, numerous Web sites. All of this new information about natural ways to rebalance hormone and nutrition levels is encouraging the consumer to look for healing products at their health food stores and seek out physicians who recommend botanicals for therapy.

The production of specific hormones often declines with age. This can lead to a number of disorders that become generally classified as arthritis.[1] Hormone deprivation is much more common today than it was some years ago. In our grandparents' generation, people were able to obtain phytohormones and enzymatic nutrients from fresh fruits and vegetables right from the farm—sometimes the same day they were picked.

Now the story is quite different. Today's hectic pace drives us to get our foods quickly and conveniently, regardless of whether they are deficient in nutrients and phytohormones. This modern hectic lifestyle plays a major role in the onset of the age-related diseases that are beginning to show up earlier and earlier in people's lives. Let's take a closer look at how we can protect ourselves from what is now being called "deficiency disorders."

## THE BOTANICAL WAY

Since hormones "control our bodily functions, including our reproductive and immune systems and our metabolism,"[2] it seems reasonable enough that hormonal deficiencies can lead to a weakened immune system. To correct this weakness, we need to answer the question, How do we find the hormone supplements we need in a plant-based form? Some years ago Russell Marker, a chemistry professor, discovered how to obtain one of these essential hormones, progesterone, from a wild yam plant named *Dioscorea mexicana*. He found he could transform one of its components, diosgenin, into progesterone.

"Yams make up the genus *Dioscorea* of the family Dioscoreaceae. There are 615 variations of *Dioscorea*, but only three are used commercially for humans . . . The name *yam* is commonly but incorrectly applied to varieties of the genus containing the sweet potatoes".[3] *Dioscorea villosa* has been found to be one of the most potent and effective yams and has been used as folk medicine in southern parts of North America for many years. Roots of the plant were boiled and made into a preparation to relieve pain from childbirth. Other cultures also used this remedy (a steroidlike substance) for muscle spasms and rheumatism.[4]

Today, natural compounding pharmacies (which sell and/or manufacture natural hormones) are using both soybeans and wild yams to convert their sterols into pregnenolone, progesterone, DHEA (dehydroepiandrosterone), estrogen, testosterone, and cortisone.[5] These hormones in their natural state can be beneficial in maintaining our health and rebalancing our hormone levels as we age. However, if the chemical structure of these substances has been changed so that they are different from that which is produced in our own body, they no longer have the same effect. They are something else dispensed under a prescriptive name.

These synthetic hormones will not produce the same physiological benefits, and they can indeed be detrimental in the long run. John R. Lee, M.D., gives a short explanation of what takes place in the laboratory to keep the molecule in its natural form: "The final product of this laboratory processing produces molecules identical to the ones found in the human body and thus, even though they are manufactured in the laboratory, we can call them natural hormones. It is unfortunate that the pharmaceutical companies then change the natural molecules to create synthetic drugs not found in nature to increase their profits at the expense of your health."[6]

These synthetic drugs (some of which are the NSAIDs) are given for the treatment of joint and back pain, heart disease, premenstrual syndrome, menopause, diabetes, osteoporosis, and other ailments. Prescriptions are written out every day for them and they are supplied by our convenient drugstores. Patients are made aware of their short-term side effects, but they don't always realize that the long-term effects can include inflammatory disorders such as arthritis.[7] There is a safer and more natural way to correct an imbalance without having to face the grave outcomes associated with drug therapy, synthetic hormone replacement, and other invasive treatments.

*The Natural Pharmacy*, written by some of the leading experts in the field of health, informs us that diosgenin, the saponin found in the wild yam, accounts for the yam's anti-inflammatory activity and other health benefits.[8] According to *The Nugent Report*, "oral *Dioscorea* crosses the mucosal cell lining of the intestines and enters the bloodstream as diosgenin."[9] Diosgenin, the sterol within wild yam, can decrease cholesterol concentration in the liver, lower blood pressure, and aid in adrenal function.[10] Studies show that dioscoran, an alkaloid isolate from

*Dioscorea villosa*, lowers the blood sugar in diabetic mice.[11] Dr. Nugent recommends it to all his diabetic patients[12] because it reduces the need for insulin.[13]

Some labs have reported that *Dioscorea* also assists in the body's utilization of progesterone.[14] A number of studies document how it reduces fat mass while simultaneously increasing lean muscle mass.[15] Additionally, it has been shown to increase bone density, restore balance to the body, and aid in antioxidant activity.[16]

The way *Dioscorea* affects joint health is demonstrated in another study that showed that standardized oral *Dioscorea* had anti-inflammatory properties.[17] Dr. Nugent has seen astounding results with conditions such as rheumatoid arthritis, fibromyalgia, and myositis. Lab tests have demonstrated that these hormones (progesterone, pregnenolone, DHEA, estrogen, testosterone, cortisone, and many more) affect each individual cell in our body.[18] These results could be why "50% of the raw material needed for steroid synthesis is provided by *dioscorea villosa*."[19]

To illustrate his point, Dr. Nugent gives us a little history of the *Dioscorea villosa* plant. It is known that it was used as food for slaves aboard the ships coming to the New World from Africa. Living in their own waste for months on the turbulent seas, many of them became ill or died. Among those who survived, many had nothing else to eat but *Dioscorea villosa*. Health benefits were noted at the time. For instance, many people's cases of rheumatism simply disappeared.[20] Dr. Nugent believes it was the phytochemicals within the plant that produced such therapeutic effects.

This might have been one of the first recorded incidents of the benefits of this substance. Since then the evidence has accumulated until its efficacy is no longer in question. Yet many in the "establishment" continue to almost categorically discount the use of *Dioscorea*. Perhaps more evaluation is in order before it's completely written off—except as a source for U.S.P. (United States Pharmacy) progesterone.

## COMPLEMENTARY AID TO A HOLISTIC LIFESTYLE

When arthritis, or any disease, strikes, we need to ask ourselves some pertinent questions: Do we need to use drugs that mask the symptoms of our deficiency disorders? Are low levels of pregnenolone exaggerating arthritic pain, memory loss, and endocrine imbalance? Are low levels of progesterone causing osteoporosis, depression, cardiovascular disorders, and joint disorders? Are high levels of estrogen causing cell proliferation, weight gain, and joint pain? Or are high levels of estrogen causing cancerous cell growth (tumors), endometriosis, fibrocystic breast disease, and poor vision? Are low levels of DHEA amplifying symptoms of diabetes, fatigue, and bone loss?

As we discussed previously, proper nutrition clearly plays a major role in maintaining health and helping the body heal itself. Choosing organic foods, natural hormones,[21] and vitamin supplementation is essential in today's world to fight environmental pollutants that end up in our food, air, and water. Some of these pollutants are known as estrogenic-mimicking toxins, which are actually "endocrine disrupters" that have been found to block our hormone receptors,[22] resulting in grave health problems.

A combination of natural therapies, including phytochemicals and phytohormones, can, however, counteract these environmental obstacles. There seems to be no end to the number of documented studies that establish the need and effectiveness of rebalancing hormonal and nutritional levels as an aid in fighting degenerative diseases. First we need to learn how our hormones affect each other negatively when out of balance and positively when in balance.[23] Then we need to apply sensible solutions to our specific needs. As an example of the importance of hormone balance and its relationship to arthritis, let's take a look at one of the many cousins of arthritis, fibromyalgia.

While searching for answers, I coincidentally met a group of people who have been diagnosed with fibromyalgia. I had no idea such a large population suffered from this disease. Because of the frequent use of the term *fibromyalgia*, I started reviewing literature about its relationship to neuromuscular problems. It turns out that fibromyalgia is one of many poorly understood conditions that has been misdiagnosed as Lyme disease.[24] In fact, it's considered one of "the most common forms of acute and chronic rheumatism."[25] Shooting and burning pain, stiffness, insomnia, and even temporomandibular joint (TMJ) syndrome are just some of the numerous characteristics of fibromyalgia, which is considered to be a rheumatic disorder.[26]

Through my own study, as well as personal experience with this group of symptoms, I also discovered that low progesterone levels and high estrogen levels have been found to be major causes of fibromyalgia, as well as other problems relating to neuromuscular disorders.[27] Progesterone helps the body maintain function and homeostasis.[28] However, when pharmaceutical companies convert the natural hormone into synthetic progestins, glucocorticoids, and estrogens, for example, the altered molecule no longer has its safe and stabilizing power.[29]

In the 1950s it was discovered that phytoprogesterones (progesterone-like materials) "were found in thousands of plant varieties."[30] Plants such as the soybean contain a sterol called stigmasterol, and the wild yam plant contains the sterol diosgenin. Both plants are commonly used to make progesterone. The sterols from these plants are converted in the lab to a molecule that naturally duplicates the progesterone activity that's normally produced in the ovaries.

Dr. Raymond Peat and A. L. Soderwall tell us that progesterone protects us at the cellular level against the effects of toxins and stress.[31] Dr. Peat found that when progesterone was combined with natural vitamin E solutions, a profound biological compatibility occurred, "increasing by as much as 2,000% progesterone's already dramatic effects." This combination was thus found to be beneficial in the treatment of a variety of problems, including autoimmune diseases, habitual miscarriages, cancer, and so much more.[32]

Dr. Peat has found that many forms of arthritis tend to "disappear" when women become pregnant.[33] This is especially interesting in light of the fact that when the placenta takes over during the last three months of pregnancy, the production of progesterone rises to 300–400 mg per day.[34] This amount is about 10 times higher than what's normally produced by an ovulating woman. What great protection progesterone provides us during pregnancy! It's the hormone that is essential for the survival of the embryo. Perhaps it's also essential for the survival of our good health.

## PROGESTERONE FOR BONE AND JOINT HEALTH

As far back as 1934, it was reported that pure crystalline progesterone was beneficial in the treatment of diseases such as arthritis and cancer. It had also been successful in treating infertility, preventing miscarriage,[35] and even reversing osteoporosis.[36] This latter disease often occurs after hormone levels of progesterone have been low for many years.

Progesterone works directly with osteoblastic, or bone-forming, cells, and as such it is the hormone responsible for building bone mass. Other studies demonstrate similar remarkable advantages in the promotion of bone formation or reduction of bone loss, thus decreasing the risk of osteoporosis.[37] As you can see, there are a variety of physiological benefits when this plant-based progesterone is taken as a supplement along with a balanced, nutritious diet.

Many holistically minded health care practitioners are now employing transdermal progesterone to prevent osteoporosis. They're finding that the use of this cream is complementary to the other care they provide their patients. A case in point was demonstrated in one patient who had signs of early osteoporosis and arthritic pain: "A 72-year-old female patient was seen on 1/11/93 . . . a bone density study revealed her bone mineral content to be abnormal. . . . [B]one width was 0.579. . . . She was placed on a topical liquid progesterone 1 ml daily for two months. After that time, she was treated with 1 ml daily for three weeks, one week of rest, and then the treatment was repeated each month thereafter in this manner. On 6/24/95 a repeat bone density study was performed and her numbers were now 0.646 or a bone density that could be compared to age 63. . . . All of her symptoms had subsided, and in fact, she has more strength and stamina than she has had in many years."[38]

Another patient, a sixty-year-old man, was diagnosed with osteoporosis. His bone density study was 0.769. After four months of receiving topical progesterone in the dosage described above, his bone density improved to 0.850.[39]

Progesterone has also been found to lower LDL cholesterol and aid in elevated blood pressures, heart disease, and even thyroid dysfunction. It has been established that hypothyroid symptoms are similar to those of arthritis.[40] And the true value of progesterone, in addition to these and many other benefits, is that it has no known side effects.[41]

It is truly rewarding to hear from women who tell me about their experiences with natural progesterone and how it has enhanced the quality of their lives. One lady in her seventies called from Montana to tell me that she'd been on Premarin, a synthetic estrogen, for twenty-three years. She was very frustrated because she suffered from the very conditions that her estrogen replacement hormone was supposed to prevent—joint pain and bone loss, which eventually led to acceleration of her osteoporosis. She also had suffered from two heart attacks.

After reading *The Estrogen Alternative*, she started using natural progesterone, not the synthetic progestins, and was thrilled when even her fibromyalgia symptoms began to disappear. The wonderful stories I continue to hear encourage me to write and explain why deficiency disorders and imbalances, whether hormonal or nutritional, don't have to be labeled with a medical diagnosis such as fibromyalgia, arthritis, or any other inflammatory disease.

## PROGESTERONE'S ROLE IN ARTHRITIS

Women suffering from fibromyalgia or from localized pain in the knees, shoulders, or hips report that the discomforts in their joints subsided significantly when they began using progesterone.[42] This is an important factor to consider when treating arthritic conditions. Dr. Lita Lee's studies confirm that taking natural progesterone can help relieve miserable muscular aches, shin splints, and arthritic pain.[43] Dr. Raymond Peat speaks about how this hormone has been found to be useful when applied topically for "inflamed tendons, damaged cartilage, or other inflammations."[44]

Dr. Peat writes that fasting is quite helpful for relieving arthritic disorders, and he goes on to say that "bacterial toxins and antigens interact with hormones and the immune system, and intestinal health should be considered as an integral part of hormone therapy."[45] This is a reminder that arthritic disorders not only involve the joints, but are systemic in nature. Looking at the overall picture by addressing hormone imbalance with progesterone, pregnenolone, or DHEA can also make a significant difference. Restoring normal levels of any one of these hormones eliminates the terrible toxic effects of conventional medicine. "Rheumatoid arthritis, osteoarthritis, lupus, scleroderma, and a variety of other 'autoimmune' diseases and connective tissue diseases respond well to these hormonal treatments."[46]

Osteoporosis has been found to occur in some women in their thirties and forties, or "five to twenty years prior to menopause." And this, of course, depends on many other factors including, but not limited to, dietary and environmental considerations.[47] It starts later in men, usually around the age of sixty.[48] (The decrease of testosterone in men may be followed not only by bone loss, but fatigue, irritability, and depression as well.)[49]

In my many conversations with women about progesterone, I have heard over and over about the benefits they have experienced—everything from the disappearance of uncomfortable fibroids to improved energy and a better outlook on life. The thought that comes to mind is: "Moms, tell your daughters what your doctors may not have told you." Having a daughter of my own was all the more reason to write about how botanical medicine can aid in disease prevention. And remember, there's a vast amount of information out there that is still not available from mainstream medicine.

Sharing what we know with friends and loved ones will allow us to participate in an important change in the prevailing practices in the health care field. And the more we take action, the greater the chance that natural alternatives will enrich our life, the lives of those we love, and perhaps many strangers we'll never even meet.

## LOW DHEA LEVELS CAUSING ARTHRITIS

DHEA is a hormone that's produced in the adrenal glands as well as in other places in the body. Etienne-Emile Baulieu was the first chemist to discover DHEA. Baulieu showed that it was made from the parent hormone pregnenolone.[50] Peter Casson, M.D., says those taking DHEA are less likely to get adult-onset diabetes than the general population.[51] And taking DHEA may also be effective in treating many forms of arthritis, including rheumatoid arthritis,[52] in people with low DHEA levels.[53] Dr. Davis Lamson found that it may relieve arthritic symptoms such as pain and morning stiffness, and it "often reduces the need for anti-inflammatory medication."[54] For this reason, hormone replacement therapy for the elderly "whose serum DHEA levels have declined substantially," might well be appropriate.[55] William Regelson, M.D., also explains that it will assist in the "metabolizing or utilizing of food," and this is important for the elderly who are not active and are prone to weight gain.[56]

Many doctors in the field of rheumatology are seeing wonderful results with patients who are suffering from lupus. Ronald F. Van Vollenhoven, M.D., Ph.D., gave his patients DHEA for approximately one year with dosages ranging from 50 to 200 mg, depending on the patient's condition. This program was a great success. It remarkably improved patients' symptoms. Other studies showed that DHEA affected immune system response by increasing both interleukin-2 and T cell production.[57]

Women in Japan suffering from lupus were reported to have had exceptionally low DHEA levels.[58] We are also hearing that, as a general rule, fibromyalgia patients have low levels of DHEA. Once these patients were placed on DHEA treatments, they had more energy and were able to resume regular exercise.[59] One report states that twenty-eight women who had a variety of lupus symptoms were given DHEA for three months and their improvement was superior to that of the patients on the placebo.[60] A study reported in the journal *Arthritis and Rheumatism* revealed similar results.[61]

Dharma Singh Khalsa, M.D., says that as we age and our DHEA level declines, degenerative diseases such as arthritis and arteriosclerosis often surface.[62] His program focuses on preventing these diseases by lowering cortisol levels and reducing mental stress. He also recommends exercise in the morning "when the glandular system is first secreting."[63]

According to researcher Joe Glickman, Jr., M.D., as we age this hormone "dramatically decreases by 80-90%" after the age of twenty.[64] This brings on many age-related diseases.[65] DHEA aids in many areas of organ health, reduces atherosclerosis, heart disease, and strokes, and supports the immune system.[66] It's been found that when "DHEA is low, the immune system cells in the gut are dysfunctional."[67] Also, DHEA significantly protects against viral infections.[68] This last point is important because there is evidence that a variety of arthritic conditions may be caused by an obscure, or unspecified, virus.[69]

It's not wise, though, for young people, especially those under thirty, to take DHEA. Doing so could very likely suppress the natural production of the hormone.[70] Another caution comes from the studies that suggest possible oxidative stress on the liver when using DHEA. However, it has also been found that taking vitamin E simultaneously may reduce this side effect and serve as a protection to the liver.

For people who are overweight, DHEA may improve liver function, since an obese person normally has a weakness in the liver.[71] Dallas Clouatre, Ph.D., reports that "very large doses of DHEA can apparently block or even reverse the influence of the genes responsible for obesity and diabetes in experimental animals."[72] So DHEA works to either use fat for energy or excrete it.

Although my personal DHEA saliva tests were found to be on the low side, I am extremely cautious about taking DHEA on a daily basis. There's no doubt that hormones such as DHEA and melatonin need to be studied more thoroughly to determine the long-term effects of supplementing it.[73] DHEA is manufactured in the body by pregnenolone.[74] Knowing this, I thought it wiser to take the parent hormone, which has the ability to manufacture all the other hormones when needed.[75] This proved for me to be the better choice.

## ESTROGEN OVERLOAD

We have previously discussed the fact that dysfunction of the endocrine system is an underlying cause of arthritis.[76] Furthermore, autoimmune disorders frequently appear when women's progesterone levels decline significantly compared to estrogen levels. The onset of thyroid problems, and even goiter, seems to be related to high estrogen and low progesterone levels.[77] An important clinical question concerning arthritis is posed by Dr. John Lee: "Is this an unrecognized symptom of estrogen toxicity . . . ?"[78] Based on the studies, this rhetorical question should pose a challenging consideration to medical science.

Problems may arise for women taking conjugated estrogens with medroxyprogesterone acetate (MPA), one of the many combinations of the more common synthetic hormones. Too many women, including myself, have been fooled by the temporary relief of symptoms that occur at the very beginning of such treatment. This imitation hormone is not dealing with possible future disorders. In fact, its long-term use may promote a host of unwanted side effects that show up in diverse ways in the postmenopausal population. It should be examined with great caution.

We really need to look a lot closer at the ramifications of this hormone called estrogen. It is not all it is heralded to be. Scientific studies are certainly not in agreement with the orthodox medical attitude toward hormone replacement therapy. The advertising campaigns from pharmaceutical commercials concerning the need for estrogen supplementation are not only misleading, but can also lead to mistreatment and to dangerous side effects. Dr. Peat reports that estrogen "tends to deprive all tissues of an adequate supply of oxygen." According to Dr. Peat, "the 'energy' it provides isn't protective." He goes on to tell us that it may activate "brain pathways that involve potentially deadly over-excitation," and can even be responsible for the "aging and death of brain cells."[79] This is one reason why estrogen has been found responsible for a variety of autoimmune diseases in particular patients, including osteoarthritis and rheumatism.[80] As for estrogen's effect on bone, animal studies now show that "estrogen retards the growth of cartilage."[81]

It is interesting to note that under federal law, we need to get a doctor's prescription to take a drug that in the end is potentially harmful. Estrogen is widely prescribed to women. Yet it is known to cause both cancer[82] and arthritic conditions.[83] Dr. Peat comments on this philosophy in a humorous yet cautionary way. He says that people who look for alternative sources of estrogen are like people who are looking for alternative forms of plane crashes. He relays a story about three women who were on estrogen: "One developed an extreme case of rheumatoid arthritis, which got worse with each dose of estrogen and disappeared when she stopped using it. Another woman had a mental breakdown within an hour of her estrogen injection and was hospitalized for six months. Her daughter began using the contraceptive pill, and died of a stroke at the age of twenty-eight. It was clear to me that estrogen had harmful effects, and that it was being promoted without adequate warnings."[84]

Dr. John Lee, citing a study from *Arthritis and Rheumatism*, states that "women who had previously used oral contraceptives were 40 percent more likely to have the immune disorder lupus . . . than women who had never used them. In fact, the incidence of all the autoimmune diseases is increased in pill users."[85] And there's much more. Other research has found estrogens to cause breast cancer, rheumatoid arthritis, heart disease, strokes, and many other serious problems.[86] On the other hand, progesterone plays an important role in reducing the flare-ups of lupus.[87]

Estrogen dominance is quite prevalent these days and it is clear that the combination of high estrogen and low progesterone levels creates many serious health problems such as osteoporosis, endometrial bleeding, and overstimulation of breast tissues.[88] If a woman is experiencing what is medically called a "luteal phase failure," which means she is not producing enough progesterone in the second half of her cycle (after ovulation), bone and joint health can be threatened.[89]

We have learned that to provide protection from the detrimental consequences of estrogen, especially when a woman's level of estradiol is high, or over 1 pg/ml (in a saliva test), progesterone levels should be about 200 times higher (0.2 ng/ml) during this phase.[90] A woman can be aware that she has a luteal phase deficiency if she is experiencing irregular or no periods, heavy bleeding, basal temperature variations, or abnormal lab work, and she can treat it with supplements of natural progesterone as opposed to synthetic progestins. This will prevent high estrogen levels from taking over during either the first part (follicular phase) or the second part (luteal phase) of the cycle, that is, before and after ovulation.

As we have mentioned, progesterone stimulates the growth of bone mass and is essential in opposing the stimulatory effect of estrogen when treating breast and uterine cancer.[91] So, it may be that simply correcting a common hormonal imbalance or deficiency is an effective solution to many ailments such as autoimmune diseases, and at the same time it may aid in glandular function.

## MYELIN SHEATH PROTECTION THROUGH HORMONES

We're finding that combinations of a variety of hormones, rather than just one individual hormone, may be what's needed for immunological and even neurological balance when combating arthritis.[92] In 1995 it was discovered that the hormone pregnenolone was essential in the healing process of damaged nerves.[93] It is also thought to have a stimulatory action on the neurotransmitter glutamate, which directly affects nerve cells.[94]

Pregnenolone declines as we age. When supplemented from natural sources, it is considered safe, with no known side effects. Even at high doses, it is transformed to multiple steroid and neurosteroid compounds, including DHEA. Billie Sahley, Ph.D., reports that it provides adrenal support and assists in the repair of the myelin sheath.[95] (The myelin sheath is the membrane protecting the brain and nervous system.)[96]

The formation of the myelin sheath occurs with the assistance of progesterone manufactured by the Schwann cells from pregnenolone. Progesterone prevents nerve trauma, short-circuiting, and chemical erosion. However, a deficiency of progesterone in these cells damages myelin formation during nerve restoration.[97]

The Schwann cells can no longer protect the myelin sheath when synthetic hormones such as oral contraceptives and the intrauterine device interfere with the progesterone receptor sites. Some disorders resulting from nerve transmission breakdown are muscle weakness, vision disorders, Parkinson's disease, diabetic neuropathy, and multiple sclerosis, among many others.[98] Progesterone may someday be the major treatment in these myelin deficiency diseases.[99] Needless to say, supplementing progesterone can be helpful for many functions in our body.[100] Betty Kamen, Ph.D., puts it this way: "The myelin sheath is to nerves what plastic insulation is to electrical wires."[101] Experiments showed that when there was nerve damage, progesterone was at the site, resulting in "a significant increase in the thickness of new myelin sheaths."[102] This was exciting news for researchers, especially when they discovered the role of progesterone in aiding myelin formation. For more information on pregnenolone and its relationship to the nervous system, refer to "Key Role for Pregnenolone in Combination Therapy that Promotes Recovery After Spinal Cord Injury" by Lloyd Guth et al., and another study entitled "Progesterone Synthesis and Myelin Formation by Schwann Cells: A Newly Demonstrated Role of Progesterone," by Schumacher M. Koenig.[103] There appears to be evidence that pregnenolone is the "long-sought-after drug that can reverse paralysis in victims of spinal cord injuries,"[104] as well as improve motor function.[105]

## PREGNENOLONE AND ITS USE IN ARTHRITIS

Let's go back to 1940 when it was discovered that pregnenolone worked safely and quite successfully in relieving rheumatoid arthritis. Some of the studies covered the effects of pregnenolone on rheumatoid arthritis. No bad effects were seen at a dosage as high as 500 mg/day.[106] Decades ago researchers found that patients suffering from arthritis reported less fatigue and pain when taking pregnenolone and at the same time showed an increase in physical strength.[107] Doctors who prescribed "300 mg of preg[nenolone] daily for forty days to patients suffering from rheumatoid arthritis" during the 1950s found similar results.[108]

In 1944, a time when natural substances were more likely to be used, pregnenolone was quite effective in hormone replacement for those who suffered degenerative diseases. Even today some medical advisers are admitting that "pregnenolone appears to have considerable potential, including possible applications to patients with memory loss, rheumatoid arthritis, fatigue, depression and premenstrual syndrome."[109] Pregnenolone is also a precursor to the release of various pituitary, adrenal, and thyroid hormones.[110]

With so many people suffering from arthritis, it's sad that the public is not informed about the number of remarkable physiological benefits derived from pregnenolone. Research has found that pregnenolone can relieve the devastating effects of systemic and neurological disorders. As the result of a study in 1995 at the University of Bordeaux in which the sciatic nerves (the large nerves extending from the end of the spine down the legs) were severed, scientists determined that both pregnenolone and progesterone had significant healing powers when nerve damage had occurred. Ray Sahelian, M.D., documents the results of this study in his book, *Pregnenolone*: "When preg [pregnenolone] and progesterone were administered, the myelin sheaths formed normally."[111] The fact that both these hormones are "significantly involved in the healing process of damaged nerves,"[112] may encourage more doctors to look at the research that addresses devastating disorders with the use of naturally occurring substances that are often found to be deficient in the body. In multiple sclerosis, for instance, the myelin sheath that protects the nerves breaks down, resulting in weakness, loss of muscular coordination, and much more. We can be grateful to medical investigators such as Dr. Sahelian and others whose research provides hope for those suffering from devastating nerve disorders such as multiple sclerosis and even the relentless pain associated with sciatica and other neurological arthritis disorders.

Ray Sahelian also reports: "A fair proportion of rheumatoid arthritics receiving preg [pregnenolone] in sufficient dosage, for an adequate period, show symptomatic changes sufficiently favorable to warrant further study. The substance has an extraordinarily low order of toxicity."[113]

A study reported in the *Journal of the American Medical Association* cites the use of pregnenolone in treating rheumatoid arthritis. Pregnenolone was selected because of "its possible role as a precursor of more active steroid hormones . . . its effect on decreasing fatigue . . . its sparing action on the adrenal cortex . . . its lack of toxicity in both animals and man," and its value to those suffering from abnormal and inflammatory joint function.[114]

The people who took part in the study all had slight cartilage disease, bone disease, or both, or abnormal joint function and inflammation. Some had suffered from their condition for four months, others for twenty-nine years. The ages ranged from thirty-one to seventy-four years. Patients were given 100 mg tablets of pregnenolone for approximately six weeks. Most patients noticed benefits in varying degrees within days. They reported diminished pain, disappearance of tenderness, greater joint mobility, less spasticity, greater strength, and the ability to climb stairs and stoop to tie their shoes. At the conclusion of this study, the patients continued to show recuperative powers in these areas.[115] Other works substantiate these findings.[116]

As explained in his book, Dr. Sahelian starts his patients on 2 to 5 mg.[117] Some patients who took 10 mg still experienced stiffness and swelling, but when the dosage was raised to 20 mg they felt relief.[118] Some find it more effective if it is used in conjunction with DHEA or other antioxidants.[119] Needless to say, it's important to eat wholesome foods when taking pregnenolone or any natural hormone.

Pregnenolone is an overlooked remedy. What William Regelson, M.D., and Carol Colman say is a "kinder and gentler treatment for arthritis"[120] deserves further investigation—perhaps even for conditions such as Alzheimer's disease. This forgotten hormone could be of great value because "pregnenolone is a substance for which the body has the enzymatic machinery to handle and is unlikely to have adverse effects."[121]

Unfortunately most doctors just don't prescribe pregnenolone instead of anti-inflammatories, cortisone, and so on. As a result some self-motivated patients have decided to pursue their own program of what could be termed self-help, or even self-survival.

I personally varied my own usage on a trial and error basis until I finally obtained optimum results. I don't suggest that for everyone. It's always better to have expert counsel. Experience did teach me, though, that each of us is an individual possessing unique biochemistry. It's our responsibility to be in tune with abnormal symptoms and our right to try to make every effort to find natural ways to prevent disease.

Dr. Sahelian has written that even though pregnenolone levels can be measured in blood or saliva tests, such tests do not tell the whole story. Not only is pregnenolone metabolized into other hormones, but it is also needed itself in every tissue and cell throughout the body. And because each person has unique capabilities of converting pregnenolone into all the steroid hormones, measurement of the precise level is not reliable.

The need for pregnenolone by the body may also vary depending on overall health of an individual or even the time of the month the dosage is taken. Some of us may require higher doses than others depending on age, sex, weight, nutritional intake, and the state of our physical as well as mental health. Even our own fluctuating state of health may warrant a change in dosage from time to time. Because of all these limiting and complex factors in evaluating accurate levels, most physicians don't normally prescribe expensive pregnenolone tests.[122]

## PREGNENOLONE VERSUS CORTISONE

Although pregnenolone was a success in the early 1940s, research on the hormone was not pursued very aggressively. Pregnenolone is a natural substance and can't be patented. Since the pharmaceutical industry did not see any significant financial return from producing it, they turned instead to synthetic cortisone. And cortisone worked. The patients were getting overnight relief, although most had no idea what was in store for them in later years when some adverse side effects kicked in. As Paavo Airola so aptly reminds us, the remedy became worse than the disease. But cortisone sales produced great profits and this became the miracle drug of choice. The adverse effects came later. No one foresaw that cortisone's short-term benefit could be at the cost of harmful effects such as softening of bones, mental disturbances, degeneration of nerves, cataracts,[123] hypertension, metabolic problems utilizing fats and protein, fluid retention, strain on the heart and kidneys,[124] debilitating effects on the immune system, decreased bone mass,[125] and susceptibility to carcinogenesis.[126]

## PREGNENOLONE SYNTHESIZED FROM CHOLESTEROL

As we discussed in chapter 4, cholesterol plays an essential role in hormone balance. Those readers suffering from arthritis may be interested to know that the hormone pregnenolone "is made from cholesterol!"[127] Unfortunately, the public is bombarded with misinformation about cholesterol, much of it from food industry ads. But once we study the body's need for good sources of this food, and become a little wiser about the function it plays in our metabolism, we begin to understand that we may be gravely depriving ourselves of the very substance we need to help sustain and balance our hormones.

Without cholesterol we would, and often do, have many problems associated with hormone deficiency. I felt it critical to stress the importance of dietary cholesterol earlier (see chapter 4) because the body's production of all steroidal hormones stems from cholesterol.

The brain has the capacity to use cholesterol to make pregnenolone. Dr. Sahelian reports, "There are enzymes in cells that convert cholesterol to preg[nenolone]. . . . The amount of preg[nenolone] made depends on how much cholesterol is brought to the mitochondria."[128] (Mitochondria are little factories in the cells where steroids are produced.) Dr. Sahelian tells us that drugs prescribed to combat high cholesterol can block the enzyme activity that's required to make pregnenolone from cholesterol. These drugs can thus cause a decline in pregnenolone. So when drugs are prescribed to lower cholesterol, other important hormones may suffer.[129]

Nevertheless, in using pregnenolone replacement the body's innate wisdom will decide which steroidal path to follow. This is because pregnenolone is the first hormone in the chain of steroid hormones that our body produces.[130] It is the building block used to manufacture all the other steroid hormones. There are two pathways that descend from pregnenolone in this process. See the following illustration. One path consists of progesterone, cortisol, and aldosterone; and the other path consists of DHEA, androstanedione, estrogens, testosterone, and other androgens. There are other metabolic compounds that are made from pregnenolone, but for simplicity's sake we will not address those here.

The main point is that using naturally occurring substances for hormone replacement turns out to be a sensible treatment and even complementary to other natural methods; it enables an injured system to reorganize and effectively recover. Pregnenolone does this by "giving rise to the greatest number of other steroids, substances that are known to facilitate coordinative processes within and among neural, metabolic, and immune systems."[131]

Hans Selye, an endocrinologist and researcher, was one of the first of the pioneers to recognize pregnenolone's numerous and valuable capabilities. Two of over thirty books that he wrote were called *Stress without Distress* and *The Stress of Life*. Isn't it interesting that he discovered the advantages of one of the hormones that reduces stress? Selye was considered by some to be "the Einstein of medicine," holding many

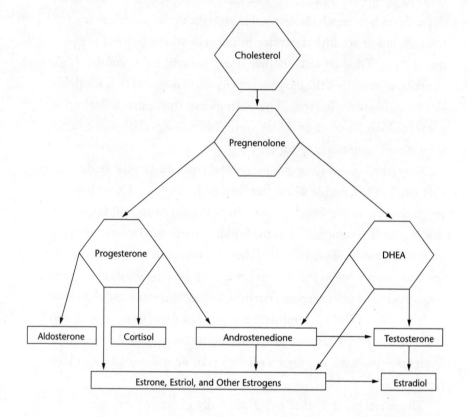

*This simplified diagram shows the conversion of cholesterol to pregnenolone. After conversion it follows two pathways, branching out to either progesterone or DHEA, from which the remaining steroid hormones are manufactured.* *

---

*Diagram information from Ray Sahelian, *Pregnenolone*, (Garden City Park, N.Y.: Avery Publishing Group, 1997), 18; Betty Kamen, *Hormone Replacement Therapy: Yes or No?* (Novato, Calif.: Nutrition Encounter Inc., 1993), 34, 42; and John R. Lee, *Natural Progesterone: The Multiple Roles of a Remarkable Hormone* (Sebastopol, Calif.: BLL Publishing, 1993), 12.

honorary degrees for his scholarly contributions. Dr. Sahelian quotes from one of Selye's scientific works: "Pregnenolone distinguishes itself from other steroids because it possesses so many different activities. Thus the compound possesses, at least in traces, every independent main pharmacological action which has hitherto been shown to be exhibited by any steroid hormone."[132]

Eugene Roberts, Ph.D., a leading expert in neurochemistry, explains that "pregnenolone and its 'offspring' may have so many facilitative effects, some of which may be achieved by giving the parent alone, and others possibly by giving the parent with one or more of the offspring."[133]

## APPROACH OF YESTERYEAR

This important and natural method for the treatment of arthritis may seem new because it is not publicly advertised in the traditional manner. But it is not really new. It has in fact been well known to doctors practicing natural alternatives for over five decades. Back then it was reported that patients with rheumatoid arthritis became pain free on pregnenolone, which was made from natural sources.[134] It was one of the first hormones shown by researchers to be beneficial.[135] Pregnenolone is not an instant cure, but when you think about it, nothing is, including supplemental vitamins and minerals. Restoring our body chemistry to obtain long-term health is the key. Anything worthwhile doesn't work overnight. Dr. Regelson says, "If you are using pregnenolone to treat arthritis, you will need to be more patient. Studies show that it can take several weeks before you will begin to feel appreciably better."[136] When it comes to bone and joint pain, bone loss leading to osteoporosis, and other degenerative diseases such as arthritis, we need to arm ourselves by looking back to a time when safer and more preventive measures were used.

Concerning deficiency diseases, however, medical doctors and even women's health periodicals still recommend estrogen for preventing bone loss. But opinions based on endocrinology studies, not those based on pharmaceutical advertising campaigns, tell us otherwise—not only about pregnenolone's and/or progesterone's benefits and estrogen's high risks, but also why these topics are not championed by the medical community.

## ARTHRITIS? OR ADRENAL BURNOUT?

All the studies we've discussed seem so sensible and easy. They allow us to finally assess our own individual needs. There's no doubt that we are faced with a challenge putting so much information to use. We could, of course, choose to ignore the problem; but if inflammatory disease hits with a vengeance, as it may, we will find frustration dominating our life. Although we can take tests that rule out some particular diseases, no tests will reveal our true needs or the state of our deficiencies.

Back when I didn't know about natural choices for systemic diseases, I had an experience that indeed frightened me. Pain dominated my every thought and deed. I could see very little hope from a future filled with pain and prescriptive drugs. My chiropractic adjustments would not hold and the pain became more severe. I was afraid of what I didn't understand. The pain was sharp and shooting and I never knew when or where it was going to strike. As my joints and body weakened, I felt any sudden motion or misstep would surely cause an injury.

During this time, I agreed to help run a children's church camp at a state park, far from any doctors or hospitals. As I started doing my very light and normally stress-free duties, I began to have a terrible time walking and even turning without sharp, shooting pains. I was terrified because I didn't know what was happening in my body, or what to do about it. The jobs I had normally found fun were suddenly stressful and torturous. I prayed hard to be temporarily relieved of my pain so that I could at least perform my job at camp. Being taken away on a stretcher to a hospital was a situation I didn't think I could handle, but I was afraid to sit or walk, so I feared it might come to that. One day the pain finally incapacitated me and it took all my energy to return to my cabin and climb up on a cot. I just collapsed on the bed, not daring to get into another position due to the discomfort.

The burning sensation in the joints became so bad that the only way I could rest without too much pain was on my back. Every time I tried to move on either side, the debilitating and brutal sensation went down my leg and to my feet. Needless to say I did not sleep much. I was terribly afraid of not being able to get out of bed in the morning.

I silently prayed. I knew prayers needed action, but what could I do? My intense plea for help reminded me that I had brought a bottle of DHEA to camp. I had had no particular intention of using it, but curiosity had prompted me to pick it up at the health store before I left. I bought it because people were raving about it, and doctors were writing books about its effectiveness. So I had put a small bottle of DHEA in my first aid kit, along with all my herbal and homeopathic remedies.

Fortunately the kit was at the head of my bed. The only thing left to do as I stared out the window at the bright stars in the black sky was reach for it. I managed to grasp it as I knocked down other items in its path. I opened it and put the drops under my tongue (25 mg). Thank goodness I had learned how much DHEA to take and how to take it while studying about natural hormone replacement for a previous book.

The next day I got up out of bed cautiously. I was weak, but miraculously I got up without help. That morning I only felt hints of sporadic discomfort, but no unbearable shooting pains. I was keenly aware that when joints, tendons, and ligaments are in such a stressed state, it's easy to fall and possibly fracture a bone.

I was fortunate that my body was sensitive, or receptive, to whatever the DHEA was doing. In spite of my frail physical condition, it was working effectively and efficiently. Regardless of the side effects I had read about, I knew by how I was feeling that I needed this adrenal boost. As a precaution, I took another 25 mg of DHEA later in the morning. As the weeks went by and I became stronger and less stressed, I began reducing the dosage to every other day. I always took my botanical progesterone along with it for balance to oppose any estrogen, testosterone, or androgens that may be kicking in from the DHEA or other environmental sources.

I never thought arthritis pain had anything to do with adrenal burnout, but after my camp experience, I learned that it certainly played a large role. As time passed, DHEA even helped my chiropractic adjustments to hold for longer periods. While going through this experience, many questions arose in my mind: Why did DHEA work so well? What does this hormone actually do for stress? Most important, what were the long-term consequences? And should DHEA only be used for extreme cases, providing temporary relief?

As I got stronger, I noticed breast pain and tenderness (signs of estrogen dominance). I later found information from *The Journal of the American Medical Association* about doctors becoming too zealous in promoting DHEA. Clinical research on animals suggest that increased serum levels of DHEA may be associated with a greater risk of ovarian and possibly prostate or other cancers.[137] And as Dr. Dean Raffelock, a clinical nutritionist, explains, "Large doses of DHEA which the body can't use are shunted into estradiol, which is exactly what we don't want."[138] Since pregnenolone is the parent hormone and seemed to be free of such adverse side effects, and considering its numerous capabilities, I found its use to be a better long-term choice for my arthritis.[139]

The decision of whether to take natural hormone replacement in the form of progesterone, pregnenolone, DHEA, or combinations of them would depend on a variety of health factors, such as age, symptoms, genetic conditions, and so on. Everybody's needs vary. With the elderly, whose diets may be poor, or with ailing individuals, progesterone alone may not be as effective in raising the body's own levels of DHEA as it would be in a healthier person. For those in their sixties and seventies, the ability to convert or metabolize natural sources of botanical hormones could certainly be less efficient than for those in their forties and fifties—depending again on one's health.

## A PERSONAL SOLUTION

My ordeal with menopause, then later with arthritis, led me to read as much as I could on these subjects. I found research that proved that botanical progesterone is as essential in dealing with premenstrual syndrome in young women as it is in helping those in menopause.[140] And sure enough, botanical progesterone got me through the throes of menopause.

I continued learning about the use of pregnenolone and its safety in alleviating joint pain. The more I read, the more confident I became as to how to appropriately use pregnenolone during times of pain or inflammation. What better way to confirm these findings than to take a plant-based source that supplied what might be deficient in my body? In a few weeks I definitely began to feel the difference. For me it proved the validity of the research on natural hormone replacement.

This course of my care turned out to be decidedly more therapeutic than a treatment employing overused, nonsteroid anti-inflammatory drugs, which have many dangerous side effects. I reflected on years past (before I knew about pregnenolone) when I too agreed to cortisone shots to treat what some doctors called bursitis, others labeled tendinitis, and still others called frozen shoulder. One orthopedic surgeon assured me of the safety of cortisone injections by saying, "I routinely give my mother cortisone shots in her shoulder once a month." At the time he had me convinced that this was a perfectly natural procedure as you get older.

Not knowing any better I thought, "If he does this for his own mother, it can't be that bad." So in my vulnerable state, I submitted to the shots, completely unaware of their potential consequences.

## OUR QUALITY OF LIFE DEPENDS ON THE CHOICES WE MAKE

So the question arises, Why haven't we heard about pregnenolone replacement, which provides so much hope for those who suffer so needlessly? As Dr. Regelson and Carol Colman state, "It is a sad fact of life that in the United States, no matter how effective a substance may be in treating illness or extending and improving the quality of life, if it is not patentable, it stands a good chance of falling by the wayside."[141]

It is time for us to find doctors who look beyond allopathic (conventional Western) medicine to those who understand the importance of using nutritional and other safe therapies such as natural hormone replacement. Unfortunately, thousands of patients, both young and old, are prescribed harsh medications that are known to have long-term detrimental effects. We can learn much by the studies on these medications and pursue better ways to help ourselves achieve optimum benefits, and in turn we can share our experiences with others. We will all gain in the end by being physically fit and being survivors of the arthritis dilemma.

## TRANSDERMAL CREAM, SUBLINGUAL, OR CAPSULE: WHICH FORM TO USE?

Many doctors are hesitant to prescribe pregnenolone or progesterone as hormone replacement therapy. Yet these two natural supplements are the ones that are synthesized from cholesterol and converted on an as-needed basis by the body into other hormones.[142] (See illustration on page 154 for the role each play in this conversion.)

Specific hormones are absorbed more efficiently when using their appropriate forms, whether it be creams (for the skin), sublinguals (for placing under the tongue), pills or capsules (to be taken orally), or others. The question then becomes: In which form should a particular hormone be taken to achieve maximum benefits?

Pregnenolone is well assimilated when taken orally or sublingually in powdered form. It dissolves well in water and, according to Dr. Raymond Peat, absorbs efficiently in the intestines and is recycled throughout the body. It lasts longer in the body than progesterone because "it improves the body's ability to produce its own pregnenolone. It tends to improve function of the thyroid and other glands, and this 'normalizing' effect on the other glands helps to account for its wide range of beneficial effects."[143]

Progesterone has been found to be effective transdermally, and this is the form recommended by many doctors practicing natural alternative therapies. Dr. John Lee says he prefers it to the pill form because the high doses that are given orally (100 to 400 mg) do not only pass through the liver, but also change into metabolites that can have unwanted side effects.[144] When applied to the skin, however, the 15 to 30 mg per day is well absorbed in target tissues, and thus can aid in what he calls "physiologic hormone balance,"[145] or, in other words, what our own body would normally produce.

Katharina Dalton, M.D., the foremost authority on PMS, confirms that the pill form is not as effective because it apparently "passes to the liver, the site of numerous progesterone receptors, where it is broken down and used, instead of being transported in the blood to the other target sites,"[146] such as the brain, nasopharyngeal passages, lungs, eyes, breasts, and lining of the womb. These are some of the areas where progesterone is needed, but unfortunately by the time oral progesterone reaches the systemic blood and brain, its concentration is quite low.[147]

For these and other reasons, Dr. Peat prefers progesterone to be taken sublingually—under the tongue—because it is more efficiently absorbed through the mucosa. Progesterone, being fat-soluble, is most effective when dissolved in vitamin E. He says it "will stimulate the ovaries and adrenals to produce progesterone" and will even energize the thyroid.

While plant-based hormones have been largely ignored by mainstream medicine, they are still available in health food stores. How satisfying it would be to find a wellness-oriented doctor who would prescribe, if needed, safe alternatives to drugs. If, however, one is self-treating, these safe supplements can be obtained from many of the manufacturers in nonprescriptive form. Most of the natural hormones can be purchased in many forms (i.e., creams, sublinguals, pills, gels, etc.) from the specialized pharmacies and manufacturers listed in appendix A. What a gift when our search for natural choices ultimately leads us to the right place.

When frightening diseases occur (arthritis, cancer, diabetes), first evaluate the possibility of a nutritional or hormonal deficiency. It may save you from the unnecessary suffering and grief that can result from misdiagnosis and mistreatment. Too often false claims about health remedies are programmed into us by those who would serve only themselves. We may be surrounded by a powerful medical establishment, but none of us should lose sight of this truth: Seeking a lifestyle that focuses on prevention of disease is still our right, opportunity, and responsibility.

# Insurance for Natural Therapies

*We can drift along with general opinion and tradition,*
*or we can throw ourselves upon the guidance of the soul*
*and steer courageously toward truth.*

**Helen Keller**

If natural therapies were covered by our insurance plans, we would be more likely to try some of the many effective holistic remedies that are available. We would also learn more about what our bodies need, and become better able to meet those needs. In the end, we would have better control over our health. As it is now, the limitations of conventional insurance plans prevent many people from taking the actions they need. Our medical expenses are typically covered only if we agree to assigned doctors, designated tests, surgery, or medications. Conservative care by a holistic practitioner is seldom completely covered. As more up-to-date diagnostic tools become available to physicians, Peter Gott, M.D., tells us, "More people are being over-treated, over-tested, over-charged—and robbed of their health in the process."[1]

The standard establishment approaches do not focus on healing. Instead they offer treatments that merely relieve the symptoms of our diseases. There's little choice but to follow the traditional allopathic path. And, as we all know, some medical doctors do not encourage us to ask questions, but to do what we're told; and to assume (hope) that the doctor knows best.

Too many people are trapped. They need help but can't get insurance for the gentler and more effective treatments that can address the root of their disorders. For most of us our insurance plans don't offer natural health care options, and it seems to be getting worse, not better.

What can we do? Can we find coverage that avoids the injustice brought on by that establishment of organized medicine: government, medical, pharmaceutical, and insurance? That would be a real challenge. But we must each do what we can to use every means available to seek healthier alternatives. It is certain that we have everything to gain and little to lose by investigating our other choices.

## ENCOURAGING MORE EFFECTIVE OPTIONS

If this were a perfect world, our insurance would cover *functional* medicine: the doctors and organizations that seek to identify the factors that trigger disease.[2] Alternative health care professions and natural treatments have been proven effective in the very areas where medicine has failed. Some of these effective choices are: homeopathy, chiropractic, naturopathy, Shiatsu, and acupuncture. If we were encouraged to try first what is natural for the body, we could avoid some of the medications that, in the end, contribute to disorders such as high cholesterol, bone loss, liver disease, and nutritional and hormonal deficiencies. The right choice could very well reduce or even eliminate the need for medication or surgery.

When I was very sick I was fortunate that my insurance policy did cover chiropractic services. If it hadn't been covered, I would probably never have discovered the benefits gained by *freedom of choice*. This choice led me to other natural health care options, the effectiveness of which I would not have recognized had I still been suffering from the chronic pain brought on by nerve interference. Unfortunately, too many others continue to suffer needlessly because of limited insurance coverage. Nor would I have been able, ultimately, to find the cure that relieved my chronic pain and crippling condition.

With health costs rising faster than inflation, more and more employers are providing health care coverage through health maintenance organizations (HMOs) or similar managed care plans. For the patient, this introduces yet another hurdle. While some of these plans may offer limited coverage for alternative care therapies, the patient does not have much control or access to them, even if the treatments are beneficial. These plans employ a "gatekeeper" approach to medicine. The patient is assigned to a primary care provider and whether the patient is allowed reimbursement for alternative care is typically left to the judgment of that physician.

## MEDICATING SYMPTOMS VERSUS PREVENTING THE CAUSE OF DISEASE

Let's reflect for a moment on the two divergent health care philosophies. The treatment we receive generally flows from one or the other conviction. The first of these concentrates on diagnosing disorders and other health-threatening conditions after they are discovered, and then attempting to cure them. This is the domain of traditional medicine. Their tools are typically surgery and drugs. To apply them, there must be a diseased body, an existing condition to be attacked. Conventional medicine has, indeed, achieved marvelous things. But far too often, its narrow reliance on the twin tools of drugs and surgery, and its custom of waiting until the problem is well established before it takes action, tend not to serve the patient well. Too often conventional medicine arrives on the scene too late, and then its actions mask the real cause of the problem, and consequently fail to eliminate it. In addition, the practitioners of conventional medicine tend to depend heavily on drug company salespeople for their education in new developments, and this often biases practitioners' judgment. Health insurance practices have grown up with this system and reflect its weaknesses and prejudices.

And the weaknesses are apparent. As stated in *Alternative Medicine* by the Burton Goldberg Group, after more than five decades of U.S. Government-sponsored research, the rate of cancer has increased in America while the death rate remains unchanged. Incredibly, the pharmaceutical-medical establishment is persecuting these "nutritionally-based cancer treatments that may be one of the keys to halting and even reversing cancerous growths."[3] Unfortunately, usual research for many diseases, including arthritis, falls under this same umbrella of organizations. This may indeed be good for business, but when it comes to health solutions, the answers are scarce and discouragingly ineffective.

Stuart Berger, M.D., writes about the "powerful ways that our medical system and its illness-centered view of medicine keeps us unhealthy ... [and] actually raises our risk of medical problems."[4] Because of this, we need to be more aware of reports in the media that contribute to public bias.

Alicia Evans, a state coordinator for Colorado-based Citizens for Health, alerts us to frequently deceptive information submitted from medical writers, including such statements as, "Casual use of natural remedies can be dangerous, experts warn." In reviewing these carefully worded phrases, she reminds us that there are no "concentrated herbal extracts that [are] as toxic as aspirin," and that "properly prescribed drugs kill at least 100,0000 people yearly."[5]

The real issue is that the efficacy of herbal remedies is posing genuine competition to pharmaceuticals. The drug companies counter, of course, by ridiculing the competition. But the public is gradually becoming more knowledgeable about preventive medicine. Their personal experiences are teaching them that benefits from what are referred to as *nutraceuticals*, are often superior to those of *pharmaceuticals*.[6]

The other approach to health care focuses on the well body (the whole body) and the ongoing task of maintaining health. Natural health care practitioners are more concerned with understanding the needs of the body and ensuring that they are provided for. Their emphasis is on the prevention of disease through good nutrition, natural supplements to restore the body's deficiencies, and other gentle natural therapies. They focus on the needs of the healthy body, including the normal changes to those requirements that come as we grow older.

In terms of insurance coverage, these natural therapies are at a disadvantage. While more and more businesses, doctors, and insurance companies are beginning to recognize the long-term advantage of spending more health care dollars on prevention, there remains the short-term problem of justifying the cost of specific therapies for insurance purposes. It is fairly easy, for example, to show that a particular malignant tissue is life threatening and that its surgical removal is vital to the health of the patient. It is far more difficult to justify the insurance costs of the natural preventive therapy that would have prevented the malignancy in the first place—even though it would almost always have cost far less.

Beyond that, of course, are the well-entrenched political and financial interests of establishment medicine lined up against the upstart natural therapies of alternative medicine. Self interest is not unknown in any area of human endeavor, much less the well-paid medical industry. But the most pernicious influence, perhaps, is that of the medical education system. As Dr. Berger tells us, *We are all at risk simply because of how our medical system functions.* Or, to put it another way, because of what our doctors didn't learn in medical school."[7] It is discouraging not to be given proper counsel and direction about the numerous natural options available and the considerable number of excellent books and comprehensive studies that explain how and why they work.[8]

It's now up to each and every one of us to act in our own way to seek answers that will improve our health, and not someone else's wallet. Although we have the freedom to speak, to worship, and to write, where is our freedom to choose a health care system that we know will work for us? The book *Alternative Medicine* includes discussion on a variety of alternative health treatments from 350 leading physicians. After hearing one patient's success story after another, it provides a reminder of the reasons to fight for our freedom to choose natural therapy—the results of which give energy to the body and the opportunity for the mind and spirit to make healthier and wiser decisions throughout life. If we don't fight, medicine will slowly, yet aggressively, become a dictator over these personal choices.

The chief executive officers, the policy makers, and all the businesses involved in traditional medicine should perhaps be reminded of the words of Benjamin Rush, M.D., one of the signers of the Declaration of Independence. In recalling his thoughts, *Alternative Medicine* heads off a chapter with a forewarning made by Dr. Rush, who was also George Washington's physician: "To restrict the art of healing to one class of men and deny equal privilege to others will constitute the Bastille of medical science. All such laws are un-American and despotic and have no place in a republic. . . . The constitution of this republic should make special privilege for medical freedom as well as religious freedom."[9]

## LOOKING TO OUR FUTURE NEEDS

The science and profession of medicine deserves applause for their many achievements and extraordinary feats. But we cannot depend on allopathic medicine alone, especially for preventive care. It must be complemented with proper nutritional initiatives: pure water, avoiding environmental pollutants, rebalancing hormone levels with botanical hormone supplementation (as needed), and many other alternative therapies. Without them we stand little chance of achieving the kind of health we need for dealing with the arduous stresses in life—especially given the deterioration of the natural environment. However, given the proper care and the right conditions, our body will usually heal itself.

I would like to share excerpts of a letter written by a close friend and cancer survivor to the president of the United States concerning the need for realistic health care reform. This woman has a family history of cancer, having lost both parents and other relatives to the disease. She herself developed breast cancer (which, incidentally, did not show up on a mammogram). Seeing her in action, I realized how individuals can exert control over their own health without succumbing to invasive, toxic, and risky procedures. She writes:

> I have had to spend a fortune out of my own pocket for nutritional supplements and other 'non-conventional' treatment, which not only saved my life but saved money by making more drastic and expensive treatment unnecessary. Please help lower the cost of health care delivery by *encouraging* alternatives . . . . Natural healing is the wave of the future! And if we would clean up our food supply, reduce the toxins in our air and water, and educate the people as to a healthy life-style, we would see sickness rates drop dramatically.

This letter undoubtedly captures the frustration of health-conscious people in today's society. And it also reminds me that I'm not alone in believing that natural therapies can withstand the pitfalls of environmental stress and people can actually overcome their genetic weaknesses. I felt the same desperation when I lost my good health and became dependent on medication and visits to my physician. Her story is reminiscent of my journey back to health through freedom of choice.

## INSURANCE, POLITICS, AND BIAS

With today's hectic lifestyle, most of us have neither the inclination nor the time to study the literature that could help solve the health problems we face daily. It takes a great deal of time and effort to seek documentation and then make intelligent decisions. Because it takes time to thoroughly understand the numerous cures for the supposedly incurable, we may instead become subconsciously influenced by the media with drug commercials endorsing "convenient toxins in brightly wrapped packages"[10] with promotion, hype, and persuasion.

But good health is worth fighting for, despite being difficult to achieve, especially when dealing with widespread bias. First of all, let's explore why health care discrimination should be illegal. The Department of Health and Human Services categorizes doctors of chiropractic as "category one" providers, along with osteopaths, medical doctors, and dentists.[11] Under the Internal Revenue Code, chiropractic care is authorized as a "medical" deduction.[12] But insurance companies inevitably put a limit on the number of office visits they'll reimburse. Obviously, there is something wrong with this system.

Here's the disparity: The same insurance companies hardly ever put a limit on the number of office visits to medical practitioners. It would seem logical that the same rules ought to apply to chiropractors. One reason for this sad state of affairs is that a number of health insurance plans and most HMOs discourage nontraditional, alternative care providers. Nor will local medical societies make an effort to refer patients to licensed health care professionals outside the medical field, even when there is an obvious affliction in the musculoskeletal area.

John McMillan Mennell, M.D., testified at the Health, Education, and Welfare hearings in Washington in 1968 that chiropractors, for instance, when dealing with musculoskeletal problems were getting patients back to work faster and at less cost than the orthodox medical practitioners. "The actuarial tables made available to the Expert Review Panel by insurance companies [during the 1968 hearings] showed that to be true."[13] One doctor writes: "No one, including organized medicine, likes to see someone else succeed where they have failed.[14] Organized medicine has spent millions of dollars to keep doctors of chiropractic from treating patients in hospitals. Yet Dr. Per Freitag, who was one of several medical doctors testifying, stated that "patients in one hospital who received chiropractic treatment are released sooner than patients in another hospital, in which he is on staff, which does not allow chiropractors."[15] Organized medicine has spent millions of dollars "working with insurance companies where they have control to keep the public from being able to receive full insurance coverage for chiropractic care." The reason why these powerful forces spend so much money "around the world each year trying to discredit chiropractic . . . is because chiropractic HAS proven to be successful for too many medical failures."[16]

It becomes a lot more personal when we hear from patients themselves, patients who did not have coverage for alternative approaches. For instance, a friend of mine, Faith, underwent major surgery twice, but she was still living with pain and multiple problems. As you listen to her testimony, understand how typical her story is and how easy it is to be swept away by mainstream medicine from natural methods that help the body heal from within. Faith talks about her experience:

> I have had every health problem from the common cold to two major operations. I have seen at least one doctor from each category listed in the Yellow Pages. My recurring problems include . . . back pain, headache, and endometriosis, along with PMS.
>
> I have been going to a medical doctor and allergist for about two years. . . . I have been suffering with back pain for a long time. In the last two years, I was hospitalized for a week and had to resume outpatient care for six months afterwards. I suffered consistently with headaches, went through numerous tests, yet found nothing. I was given all kinds of pain medication, which worked for a while but caused me to feel tired and irritable. I still had headaches, but because of the medication I was deceived into believing they were less severe.
>
> My neurological physicians could only give me medication to relieve my suffering.[17]

Faith was depressed and still in pain when she was finally introduced to her current chiropractor. She went to him in tears and was skeptical as to how this treatment could work. However, within a short period, the pain slowly began to subside. She is now better and has thrown away most of her medications. Insurance should cover such licensed doctors who can provide the assistance that Faith received.

Another instance is described in a letter to the editor of the *Atlanta Journal and Constitution:*

> The American Medical Association has led an unforgivable effort to promote ignorance of the wonderful benefits of the chiropractic profession. Countless victims of common back pain have suffered needlessly when advised by the medical profession that chiropractors were dangerous.
>
> As a victim of this cruel medical smokescreen, I was treated for back pain and leg numbness with painkillers and muscle relaxants. I was told not to go to a chiropractor. After two years without relief by the medics, desperation sent me to a chiropractic doctor. Instead of a "broken back," he gave me nearly complete relief with the very first visit!
>
> The AMA can never sufficiently pay back those of us who have suffered from their selfish unlawful misconduct. They should be forced to begin at once a massive reeducation of the public at their own expense.[18]

## THE INSURANCE RUNAROUND

In the health insurance game, it's always the patient who gets caught in the squeeze between providers and payers. Nowhere is this more common than in worker's compensation laws. If you're covered under worker's compensation, you must follow specific steps to make an appointment with a licensed doctor of your choice. You are given a list from which you are allowed to select a doctor. If your doctor is not stipulated there, you must first see a medical doctor. If there is no improvement in your condition, then another medical doctor must be seen for at least two successive appointments. If you are still in pain, authorization may then be given to see the doctor you have selected.

But all this takes time, and time is crucial when you're in distress. Your body continues to regress as more drugs are introduced to relieve discomfort. Unfortunately by this time you may be too sick to insist on receiving a referral.

Does this process sound excessive, biased, and even unjust? Most of us would find the procedure to be entirely absurd. However, in these matters our government is not governed by what is sound or even sensible for patient health. Let's look at Dr. Elliott Segal's philosophy on the prevention of crisis therapy:

> We hesitate to go to a chiropractor when our insurance does not cover such treatment. It costs a lot of money to stay healthy. When you think about it, it costs a lot of money to be sick (time away from work, expensive drugs, side effects of these drugs, frustrating doctor appointments when the problem is not found, hardship on the family). Good health does not cost, it pays and it pays.
>
> Perhaps we should consider taking some of the money that we are paying to insurance companies and use it for chiropractic care to insure that we don't get sick in the first place. . . . It seems to make more sense . . . . Now, when you go to Prudential and buy what you think is life insurance, you're not buying life insurance at all. . . . You're buying death insurance.
>
> They guarantee you that when you die somebody gets some money, which is nice, but how much nicer to insure that you have a reasonable chance of staying healthy and feeling good while you are alive by keeping the power turned on in the whole body. . . . And that is what chiropractic is all about.[19]

## THINGS WE CAN DO

Our prayers for help will be answered only when we act—when we seek what is good and effective, learn what to do, and do what we have learned is right. Change will not happen unless, and until, we make it happen. We must become activists, not passivists, in matters relating to our own health. And from there we can perhaps work on reconstructing the public's attitude toward health and disease. It is also up to us to speak out, to inspire others and protect them from exploitation.

It will be a great day in history when alternative care becomes an integral part of the existing health care system. In our endeavor to communicate the need to eliminate social injustice, the life of Victor Hugo comes to mind. Through his writing (*The Hunchback of Notre Dame*, *Les Miserables*, and many more) his words reflected the outrage of inequality: "There is one thing stronger than all the armies in the world, and that is an idea whose time has come."[20] You might want to start by looking at insurance companies that may pay for natural therapies and have programs to encourage people to take better care of themselves. For example:

Alternative Health Group:
805-734-6003 (phone), 805-379-1580 (fax)
Alliance for Natural Health:
708-974-9373 (phone), 708-974-6002 (fax)
Alternative Health Care Options:
704-523-3440 (phone), 704-523-0341 (fax)
American Western Life Insurance Company:
800-782-9200, 714-846-1413

Meanwhile, if your insurance provider does cover natural alternatives, you can take positive steps to initiate change. (1) Find out the names of your legislators on a state and national level and try to get insurance legislation introduced that improves coverage of natural alternatives. Democracy *does* work if enough people get involved. (2) Organize a national letter-writing campaign to legislators. 3) If you're self-employed, cancel your policy and tell your insurance company in writing of the reason. (4) Seek out insurance companies that do cover natural alternatives, even if it costs more, and spread the word. Any small step you take in this area will ultimately affect your health and the health of others.

The letter below is from one of my chiropractors, who wrote to my insurance company about my coverage. It shows that my case was not an isolated situation. The message could be helpful to all those insurance companies that limit their coverage to medication and surgery. There is evidently a rule that insurance companies do not cover "preventive" care. The letter points out a major inconsistency in this rule. This incongruous concept should be challenged. Feel free to use this information when formatting your own letter to your insurance company. Or you may revise this according to your needs to be sent by your doctor to your insurance company or your business that handles your group insurance.

To: [Your insurance company]
Attn.: Program Administrator for Major Medical
Address:

(Your name)_____ is a patient of mine. Please consider her/him for coverage of chiropractic care under your medical plan for the reasons listed below. My initial examinations revealed that [she/he] is in need of chiropractic care because of (condition) _____.

[Have your doctor insert her/his exam findings and treatment recommendation at this point in the letter and then perhaps note the following if you're on maintenance care.]

(Patient's name)_____ may require more frequent and intense care for short periods of time, after which she/he will probably be able to return to the normal activities of daily living with little or no symptoms. She/he can then maintain these activities with a minimal amount of care. However, the care she/he receives during these asymptomatic times is crucial to her/his health and well-being. It is this care that helps prevent the exacerbations that would ultimately occur more frequently.

Is this preventive care? It is, in the same sense as when a diabetic takes daily insulin; an asthmatic takes Proventil; a person with high blood pressure or a hypothyroid condition takes daily medication; or myriad other conditions are controlled by some form of periodic treatment. There are many varieties of preventive care. (Patient's name) chooses chiropractic care to keep her/him healthy and functional and free from pain. If she/he were taking daily doses of muscle relaxants, painkillers, and even anti-inflammatories (proven fatal at times[21]), this patient would probably be covered by her/his insurance. Unfortunately, these conventional treatments don't seem to help her/him and in addition can cause uncomfortable side effects. She/he therefore chooses to remain drug free. If or when there comes a time when the conservative treatment she/he is receiving is not working as well as it has been, she/he will probably consider another type of therapy to enhance the care she/he is receiving.

I have enclosed copies of my daily notes and recent exam findings for your review. I urge you to help (patient's name) maintain her/his health in the conservative manner she/he has chosen.

Sincerely,

(Doctor's name)

## A PERSONAL LETTER FROM YOU
## TO THE POLICY MAKERS

Write to the people in power. Send them the studies from books on naturopathic, homeopathic, chiropractic, and other gentle and effective therapies. I sent copies of my books to many policy makers telling them it's my hope that from the information it contains, they will better understand that every patient should have a moral right to select any licensed and reputable doctor of one's own choice as a *primary* health care provider. These doctors are trained to find the cause of our disorders. They do not claim to cure arthritis, allergies, immune deficiency, or other diseases. They are trained to find the root to the disorder so that the body will heal itself—without drugs. This may be performed by correcting nerve interference, discovering a chemical imbalance through kinesiology, or opening meridian pathways through acupuncture and Shiatsu to enhance energy and circulation and so forth.

This change could save us from a lot of the outrageous hospital bills and would be a constructive step in achieving good health and saving lives. The choice of alternative health care should always be available under insurance coverage, not only for the patient's sake, but for the sake of the country.

## ABOUT SECOND OPINIONS

If you have already made the rounds of medical doctors, or spent a lot of your life in and out of hospitals, and suffered well-meant but protracted and misdirected treatment that failed to bring relief, a second opinion from another medical doctor may often amount to no more than a repetition of the same diagnosis. After all, both opinions start from the same premise.

But obtaining a second opinion from a doctor in another health care profession can be different. It can provide a fresh look at the situation from a different perspective—an alternative to the allopathic view. If we pass up the chance, thinking, "My doctor knows best, I'll just go along with the recommended surgery and get it over with," we may be closing a door to better health and a better life.

A neighbor of mine may have done this. His problem began with just cramping in his leg—a circulatory problem. After various treatments, his doctor eventually recommended arterial bypass surgery. A few days after surgery complications set in and his legs became gangrenous. They had to be amputated. This was a tragic experience, and maybe an avoidable one. A second opinion from a doctor who understands the alternatives to medication and surgery might have saved my neighbor from the fate he now lives with. We'll never know, because that was a road not taken.

If second opinions from doctors who focus on natural healing were to become routine, it might also help end the persistent upward spiral in the cost of health care. Referrals to specialists in natural health care who recognize and use a conservative approach to neuromusculoskeletal problems can often circumvent a patient's experience of pre- and post-surgical trauma and its aftermath. We, the patients, have everything to gain if our physician recommends a second opinion from a specialist in another health care field who focuses on natural alternatives.

This book is dedicated to doctors who specialize in alternatives to drugs, and who have given us the confidence we need to take control of our own destiny. Unless we strive for change, the existing medical establishment will keep right on rolling, and our freedom of choice will continue to be limited. And many will continue to suffer from acute and chronic diseases that might have been eased. It's time to give priority to the alternatives: chiropractic, naturopathy, homeopathy, herbal remedies, and other preventive care. The time has come to promote a quality lifestyle that can help us to achieve both nutritional and hormonal balance when seeking optimal health.

## Epilogue

# Intercepting Hereditary Traits

There is a substantial amount of evidence that arthritis is one of the most progressively devastating diseases. And research by Jeffrey S. Bland, Ph.D., shows that "genes, environment, diet, lifestyle, and stress factors all play a role in defining the risk and progression of inflammation-related diseases."[1]

The abuse placed on the body with drugs and invasive tests, together with the substantial buildup of toxins from our polluted environment, can certainly hinder the immune system. These chemicals are recognized by the body as foreign substances that can't be utilized. The accumulation of synthetic ingredients not only obstructs the innate power of the body to heal itself, but also causes collateral damage to the human spirit.

Envision for a moment a time when we know how to combat the harmful effects of our surroundings and purge them from our mind and body. The question then arises as to whether this could affect our so-called genetic predispositions to disease. As I was reading a family biography that focused on this subject, but on a higher plane of health, I saw a correlation. It was in a prayer spoken by my grandfather:

> Lord . . . help me to know my *hereditary* evils, my *acquired* evils,
> all the evils that turn away the Divine influx from heaven . . .
> help me to get rid of them.[2]

I often meditate on these insightful words and can't help but ponder the intimate correspondence between the physical and spiritual planes.[3] Could it be that when we master the ability to refuse what is artificial and not useful to the body we may actually "rid" ourselves of some so-called congenital, but perhaps self-imposed, physical disorders? When we allow, instead, God-given live foods to do our healing, could this perfect influx from a higher order intercept genetic predisposition to disease?

## Appendix A

# Resources

## PHARMACIES

Many of the following natural compounding pharmacies are unique in that they can customize prescription medicines to meet a patient's individual requirements.

Apothecure, Inc.
13720 Midway Rd.
Dallas, TX 75244
(800) 969-6601

Bellgrove Pharmacy
1535 116th Ave. NE
Bellevue, WA 98004
(800) 446-2123

Belmar Pharmacy
12860 West Cedar Dr., Suite 210
Lakewood, CO 80228
(800) 525-9473

California Pharmacy and
    Compounding Center
307 Placentia Ave., #0102
Newport Beach, CA 92663
(800) 575-7776

Clark's Pharmacy
15615 Bel-Red Rd.
Bellevue, WA 98008
(800) 480-DHEA

Delk Pharmacy
1602 Hatchner Lane
Columbia, TN 38401
(615) 388-3952

Homelink Natural Pharmacy
381 Van Ness Ave., Suite 1507
Torrance, CA 90501
(800) 272-4767

Hopewell Pharmacy
One West Broad St.
Hopewell, NJ 08525
(800) 792-6670

Madison Pharmacy Associates
429 Gammon Place
Madison, WI 53719-9786
(800) 558-7046

Snyder-Mark Drugs Roselle
384 East Irving Park
Roselle, IL 60172
(800) PRO-GEST

Triad Compounding
1109 East Artesia Blvd., Suite H
Cerritos, CA 90703
(800) 851-7900

Trumarx Drugs
501 Gordon Ave.
Thomasville, GA 31792
(800) 552-9997

Wellness Health and
  Pharmaceuticals
2800 South 18th St.
Birmingham, AL 35209
(800) 227-2627

The Women's International
  Pharmacy
5708 Monona Dr.
Madison, WI 53716
(800) 699-8144

The Women's International
  Pharmacy
13925 West Meeker Blvd., Suite 13
Sun City West, AZ 85375
(800) 699-8143

## MANUFACTURERS AND DISTRIBUTORS

Many of the following manufacturers provide a variety of nonprescription remedies to meet your individual requirements.

AIM
3904 East Flamingo
Nampa, ID 83687-3100
(800) 456-2462

Alvin Last, Inc.
425 Saw Mill River Rd.
Ardsley, NY 10502
(800) 527-8123

Angel Care U.S.A.
3666 N. Peachtree Rd., Suite 300
Atlanta, GA 30341
(800) 235-9732

Beyond-A-Century
HC 76 Box 200
Greenville, ME 04441
(800) 777-1324

Bio-Nutritional Formulas
106 E. Jericho Tpke.
Mineola, NY 11501
(800) 950-8484

Broadmoore Labs Inc.
3875 Telegraph Rd. #294
Ventura, CA 93003
(800) 822-3712

Dixie PMS and Menopause
    Center
2161 Newmarket Parkway
Suite 222
Marietta, GA 30067
(800) PMS-9232

Easy Way International
5340 Commerce Circle, #E
Indianapolis, IN 46237
(800) 267-4522

Elation Therapy
4371 Roswell Rd.
Marietta, GA 30062
(888) 535-7632

Emerson Ecologics, Inc.
7 Commerce Drive
Bedford, NH 03110
(800) 654-4432

Health & Science Research
    Institute, Inc.
661 Beville Road #101
South Daytona Beach, FL 32119
(888) 222-1415

Health Watchers System
13402 North Scottsdale Rd.
Suite 150
Scottsdale, AZ 85254-4056
(800) 321-6917

HM Enterprises
P. O. Box 115
Norcross, GA 30091-0115
(800) 742-4773

International Health
8704 East Mulberry St.
Scottsdale, AZ 85251-5023
(800) 481-9987

International Nutrition
P.O. Box 4069
Deerfield Beach, FL 33442-4069
(800) 726-8404

Karuna Corporation
42 Digital Dr., Suite 7
Novato, CA 94949
(888) 749-8643

Kenogen
P.O. Box 5764
Eugene, OR 97405
(888) 818-5052

Kokoro, LLC
P.O. Box 597
Tustin, CA 92781
(800) 599-9412

Life-Flo Health Care Products
8126 N. 23rd Ave., Suite #A
Phoenix, AZ 85021
(888) 999-7440

Nature's Nutrition, Inc.
6425 Anderson Way
Melbourne, FL 32940
(800) 242-1115

Neways
150 East 400 North
Salem, UT 84653
(800) 998-7232

Nutraceutics Corporation
3317 N.W. 10th Terrace, Suite 404
Fort Lauderdale, FL 33309
(800) 851-7007

NutrSupplies, Inc.
P.O. Box 750
Sudbury, MA 01776
(800) 906-8874

Phillips Nutritionals
26 Commerce Center Drive
Henderson, NV 89014
(800) 514-5115

Products of Nature International
2842 Main St., P.M.B. 324
Glastonbury, CT 06033
(800) 639-2449

Pure Essence Laboratories, Inc.
P.O. Box 95397
Las Vegas, NV 89193
(888) 254-8000

Pure Health International
P. O. Box 720003
Atlanta, GA 30358
(800) 311-2186

Restored Balance Inc.
42 Meadowbridge Dr., S. W.
Cartersville, GA 30120
(800) 865-7499

Sarati International
Rt. 3, Box 385
Ted Hunt Rd.
Los Fresnos, TX 78566
(800) 900-0701

Sedna Specialty Health Products
P.O. Box 1453
Andrews, NC 28901
(800) 223-0858

Springboard
2801 Salina Hwy., Bldg. F
Monterey, CA 93940
(800) 662-8045

THG Health Products, Inc.
P.O. Box 97
Oxford, PA 19363-0097
(888) 623-4372

Transitions for Women
621 SW Alder, Suite 900
Portland, OR 97205
(800) 888-6814

Young Again Nutrients
3219 Hickory Hollow Rd.
The Woodlands, TX 77380
(877) 205-0040

# ORGANIZATIONS

To support you in your freedom of choice, the following organizations can help you with questions and your search for a doctor who practices alternative medicine in your area. In addition, this Web site should be helpful to patients and chiropractors everywhere: www.activator.com

American Association of
  Naturopathic Physicians
601 Valley St., Suite 105
Seattle, WA 98109
(206) 298-0126
www.naturopathic.org/
  findnd.html

American Holistic Health
  Association
P.O. Box 17400
Annaheim, CA 92817-7400
(714) 779-6152
http://ahha.org

American College for
  Advancement in Medicine
23121 Verdugo Dr.
Laguna Hills, CA 92654
(800) 532-3688
www.acam.org/generalpub

American Osteopathic
  Association
142 E. Ontario St.
Chicago, IL 60611
(800) 621-1773
www.aoa-net.org

Center for Holistic
  Life Extension
482 W. San Ysidro Blvd., Suite
  1365
San Ysidro, CA 92713
(800) 664-8660
www.extendlife.com

National Center for
  Homeopathy
801 North Fairfax St., Suite 306
Alexandria, VA 22314
(703) 548-7790
www.homeopathic.org

International Chiropractors
  Association (ICA)
1110 N. Glebe Rd., Suite 1000
Arlington, VA 22201
(800) 423-4690
www.chiropractic.org

American Chiropractic
  Association (ACA)
1701 Clarendon Blvd.
Arlington, VA 22209
(800) 986-4636
www.amerchiro.org

# ORGANIC MEATS

Ask the grocery store in your area to purchase meat from one of the following free-range and organic meat growers. Most of these brands of meat are free of antibiotics, growth hormone stimulants, herbicides, and pesticides. For more information contact the Organic Trade Association at (413) 774-7511.

Barry Farms Enterprises (meat, poultry)
Ohio
(419) 228-4640

Calco International, Inc. (beef, pork)
California
(510) 887-0882

Coleman Natural Products, Inc. (beef, lamb)
5140 Race Court
Denver, CO 80216
(303) 887-0882

Dale Filburn Farms (beef, pork, lamb, chicken)
Ohio
(937) 787-4885

Dixie Dreams Ranch (beef)
Louisiana
(318) 686-2760

Lasater Grasslands Beef
New Mexico
(719) 541-2855

Maverick Ranch
Idaho
(800) 497-2624

Lily & Rose Farm (lamb)
Canada
(306) 335-2210

Makinajian Poultry Farm
New York
(516) 368-9320

Mountain Meadows Farm, Inc.
Vermont
(802) 349-7344

New Mexico Organic Meat Growers (turkey, chicken, geese, ducks, beef)
New Mexico
(505) 579-4314

North Hollow Farm
Vermont
(877) 304-2333

Northwest Organic Foods (beef)
Washington
(509) 657-3400

Organic Valley/CROPP
Wisconsin
(888) 444-6455

Pahrump Heifer Ranch (beef)
California
(209) 531-9875

Peaceful Acres Farm (beef)
California
(814) 448-3132

Petaluma Poultry
California
(707) 763-1904

Sunday's Manor Farm (beef,
    chicken, goats, pheasants, rabbit)
Maryland
(301) 631-0956

Sunnyside Farm LLC (beef)
Virginia
(540) 675-2627

The Rolling Hills Farm & Ranch
    (beef, chicken, ducks)
Canada
(306) 728-3732

White Mountain Farm, Inc. (beef)
Colorado
(719) 378-243

# Appendix B

# Suggested Reading

## Diet's Effect on Arthritis

Childress, N. F. "A Relationship of Arthritis to the Solanaceae (Night-shades)." *Journal of the International Academy of Preventive Medicine* (1982): 31–37.

Darlington, I. G., et al. "Diets for Rheumatoid Arthritis." *Lancet* 338 (1991): 1209.

Deal, C. L., et al. "Treatment of Arthritis with Topical Capsaicin: A Double-Blind Trial." *Clinical Therapeutics* 13 (1991): 383–95.

Kjeldsen-Kragh, J., et al. "Controlled Trial of Fasting and One-Year Vegetarian Diet in Rheumatoid Arthritis." *Lancet* 338 (1991): 899–902.

Nenonen, M., et al. "Effects of Uncooked Vegan Food—'Living Food'—on Rheumatoid Arthritis, A Three Month Controlled and Randomized Study." *American Journal of Clinical Nutrition* (abstract 48) 56 (1992): 762.

Panush, R. S. "Possible Role of Food Sensitivity in Arthritis." *Annals of Allergy* 62 (Part II) (1988): 31–35.

Panush, R. S., et al. "Diet Therapy for Rheumatoid Arthritis." *Arthritis and Rheumatism* 26 (1983): 462–71.

Skoldstram, I., et al. "Fasting and Vegan Diet in Rheumatoid Arthritis." *Scandinavian Journal of Rheumatology* 15 (1987): 219–21.

Taylor, M. R. "Food Allergy as an Etiological Factor in Arthropathies: A Survey." *Journal of the International Academy of Preventive Medicine* 8 (1983): 28–38.

Zeller, M. "Rheumatoid Arthritis—Food Allergy as a Factor." *Annals of Allergy* 7 (1949): 200–39.

## Nutritional Healing

Balch, James and Phyllis Balch. *Prescription for Nutritional Healing*. Garden City Park, N.Y.: Avery Publishing Group, 1990.

The Burton Goldberg Group. *Alternative Medicine*. Puyallup, Wash.: Future Medicine Publishing, 1993.

Joel R. Robbins. *Health Through Nutrition*. Tulsa, Okla.: Health Dynamics, 2000.

Joel R. Robbins. *Eating for Health and Wellness*. Tulsa, Okla.: Health Dynamics, 1999.

Joel R. Robbins. *Attitudes and Health*. Tulsa, Okla.: Health Dynamics, 2000.

Joel R. Robbins. *Pregnancy, Childbirth and Children's Diet*. Tulsa, Okla.: Health Dynamics, 2000.

Joel R. Robbins. *Juicing for Health*. Tulsa, Okla.: Health Dynamics, 1999.

Walker, N. W. *Fresh Vegetable and Fruit Juices*. Ottawa, Ill.: Caroline House, 1981.

## Enzyme Support

Liebow, C., and S. S. Rothman. "Enteropancreatic Circulation of Digestive Enzymes." *Science* 189 (1975): 472–74.

Lopez, D. A. *Enzymes: The Fountain of Life*. Charleston, S.C.: The Neville Press, 1994, 227–43.

Ransberger, K. "Enzyme Treatment of Immune Complex Disease." *Arthritis and Rheumatism* 8 (1986): 16–19.

Steffen, C., et al. "Enzyme Therapy in Comparison with Immune Complex Determinations in Chronic Polyarteritis." *Rheumatology* 44 (1985).

Taussig, S. J., et al. "Bromelain: A Proteolytic Enzyme and Its Clinical Application." *Hiroshima Journal of Medical Sciences* 21 (1975): 185–93.

## Vitamin and Herb Supplements

Aihara, Herman. *Acid & Alkaline*. Brookline, Mass.: George Ohsawa Macrobiotic Foundation, 1986.

Andrecht, Venus Catherine. *The Herb Lady's Notebook*. Ramona, Calif.: Ransom Hill Press, 1992.

Bingham, R., et al. "Yucca Plant Saponin in the Management of Arthritis." *Journal of Applied Nutrition* 27 (1975): 45–50.

DiSilvestro, R. A., et al. "Effects of Copper Supplementation on Ceruloplasmin and Copper-Zinc Superoxide Dismutase in Free-Living Rheumatoid Arthritis Patients." *Journal of the American College of Nutrition* 11 (1992): 177–80.

Drovanti, A., et al. "Therapeutic Activity of Oral Glucosamine Sulfate in Osteoarthritis: A Placebo-Controlled Double-Blind Investigation." *Clinical Therapeutics* 3, no. 4 (1980): 260–72.

Foster, Steven. *101 Medicinal Herbs: An Illustrated Guide.* Loveland, Colo.: Interweave Press, 1998.

Hoffer, A. "Treatment of Arthritis by Nicotinic Acid and Nicotinamide." *Journal of the Canadian Medical Association* 81 (1959): 235–38.

Hoffman, David. *The Herbal Handbook.* Rochester, Vt.: Healing Arts Press, 1987.

Job, C., et al. "Zinc Sulphate in the Treatment of Rheumatoid Arthritis." *Arthritis and Rheumatism* 23 (1980): 1408.

Jonas, W. B., et al. "The Effect of Niacinamide on Osteoarthritis: A Pilot Study." *Inflammation Research* 45 (1996): 330–34.

Kaufman, W. "The Use of Vitamin Therapy for Joint Mobility. Therapeutic Reversal of a Common Clinical Manifestation of the 'Normal' Aging Process." *Connecticut State Medical Journal* 17, no. 7 (1953): 584–89.

Kroeger, Hanna. *Heal Your Life with Home Remedies and Herbs.* Carlsbad, Calif.: 1998.

Kulkarni, R. R., et al. "Treatment of Osteoarthritis with a Herbomineral Formulation: A Double-Blind, Placebo-Controlled, Cross-Over Study." *Journal of Ethnopharmacology* 33 (1991): 91–95.

Lee, Royal. "Vitamins F and $F_2$." *Vitamin News* (1949): 159–60.

Lininger, Skye, and Jonathan Wright, et al. *The Natural Pharmacy.* Rocklin, Calif.: Prima Health, 1998, 320.

Machtey, I., et al. "Tocopherol in Osteoarthritis: A Controlled Pilot Study." *Journal of the American Geriatrics Society* 25, no. 7 (1978): 328–30.

*Magic and Medicine of Plants.* New York: Reader's Digest Association, 1993.

Mowrey, Daniel B. *The Scientific Validation of Herbal Medicine.* New Canaan, Ct.: Keats Publishing, 1990.

Rector-Page, Linda. *Herbal Pharmacy*. Soquel, Calif.: Healthy Healing Publications, 1998.

Scherak, O. "Vitamin E and Rheumatoid Arthritis." *Arthritis and Rheumatism* 34 (1991): 1205–6.

Simkin, P. A. "Treatment of Rheumatoid Arthritis with Oral Zinc Sulfate." *Agents and Actions* 8 (supplement) (1982): 587–96.

Travers, R. I., et al. "Boron and Arthritis: The Result of a Double-Blind Pilot Study." *Journal of Nutritional Medicine* 1 (1990): 127–32.

Walker, W. R., et al. "An Investigation of the Therapeutic Value of the 'Copper Bracelet'—Dermal Assimilation of Copper in Arthritic/Rheumatic Conditions." *Agents and Actions* 6 (1976): 454–59.

## Homeopathy

Coulter, Harris. *Homeopathic Science and Modern Medicine: The Physics of Healing with Microdoses*. Richmond, Calif.: North Atlantic Books, 1980.

Ullman, Dana. *The Consumer's Guide to Homeopathy: The Definitive Resource for Understanding Homeopathic Medicine and Making It Work for You*. New York: J. P. Tarcher, 1996.

## Benefits of Pregnenolone, DHEA, and Progesterone

Coleman, D. L., et al. "Therapeutic Effects of Dehydroepiandrosterone (DHEA) in Diabetic Mice." *Diabetes* 32, no. 9 (1982): 830–33.

Davison, R., et al. "Effects of Delta 5 Pregnenolone in Rheumatoid Arthritis." *Archives of Internal Medicine* 85 (1950): 365–88.

Freeman, H., et al. "Therapeutic Efficacy of Delta 5 Pregnenolone in Rheumatoid Arthritis." *Journal of the American Medical Association* 143, (1950): 338–44.

George, M. S., et al. "CSF Neuroactive Steroids in Affective Disorders: Pregnenolone, Progesterone, and DBI." *Biological Psychiatry* 35 (1994): 775–80.

Leary, Warren E. "Progesterone May Play Major Role in the Prevention of Nerve Disease." *New York Times*, 27 June 1995, C3.

Madhu, C. "Protective Effect of Pregnenolone 16 Alpha Carbonitrile on Acetaminophen-Induced Hepatotoxicity in Hamsters." *Toxicology and Applied Pharmacology* 109 (1991): 305–13.

McGavack, T. H., et al. "The Use of Delta 5 Pregnenolone in Various Clinical Disorders." *Journal of Clinical Endocrinology* 11 (1951): 559–77.

Morales, A. J., et al. "Effects of Replacement Dose of Dehydroepiandrosterone in Men and Women of Advancing Age." *Journal of Clinical Endocrinology and Metabolism* 78, no. 6 (1994): 1360–67.

Morfin, R., et al. "Pregnenolone and DHEA as Precursors of Native Hydroxylated Metabolites which Increase the Immune Response in Mice." *Journal of Steroid Biochemistry and Molecular Biology* 50 (1994): 91–100.

## Danger of Estrogenic Hormones

Brinton, L.A., et al. "Oral Contraceptives and Breast Cancer Risk Among Younger Women." *Journal of the National Cancer Institute* 98, no. 11 (1995): 827–35.

Cavalieri, E. L., et al. "Molecular Origin of Cancer; Catechol Estrogen-3, 4-Quinones as Endogenous Tumor Initiators." *Proceedings of the National Academy of Science* 94 (1994): 10937–42.

Epstein, Samuel S. and Pat Cody. "New Drug Poses Risk of Ovarian Cancer." *Chicago Tribune*, 19 April 1998.

Fischman, J., et al. "The Role of Estrogen in Mammary Carcinogenesis." *Annals of the New York Academy of Sciences* 768, no. 91 (1995).

Rodriguez, C., et al. "Estrogen Replacement Therapy and Fatal Ovarian Cancer." *American Journal of Epidemiology* 141 (1995): 828–34.

Rose, Peter G. "Medical Progress: Endometrial Carcinoma." *New England Journal of Medicine* 335 (1996): 640–49.

Service, Robert F. "New Role for Estrogen in Cancer?" *Science* 179 (1998): 1631–33.

Veronesi, U., et al. "Prevention of Breast Cancer with Tamoxifen: Preliminary Findings from the Italian Randomised Trial Among Hysterectomised Women." *Lancet* 352 (1998): 93–97.

Yager, J. D., et al. "Molecular Mechanisms of Estrogen Carcinogenesis." *Annual Review of Pharmacology and Toxicology* 36 (1996): 203–232.

## Osteoporosis

Berengolts, E. L., et al. "Comparison of the Effects of Progesterone and Estrogen on Established Bone Loss in Ovariectomized Aged Rats." *Cells and Materials* (supplement 1) (1991): 105–11.

Berengolts, E. L., et al. "Effects of Progesterone on Post-Ovariectomy Bone Loss in Aged Rats." *Journal of Bone and Mineral Research* 5 (1990): 1143–47.

Burnett, C. C., et al. "Influence of Estrogen and Progesterone on Matrix-Induced Endochondral Bone Formation." *Calcified Tissue International* 35 (1983): 609–14.

Cummings, S. R., et al. "Endogenous Hormones and the Risk of Hip and Vertebral Fracture Among Older Women." *New England Journal of Medicine* 339 (1998): 733–38.

Grady, D., et al. "Venous Thromboembolism." *Journal of the American Medical Association* 13 (1997).

Griffiths, Joel. "Progesterone Reported to Increase Bone Density 10% in Six Months." *Med Tribune*, 29 November 1990.

Halberstam, M. J. "If Estrogens Retard Osteoporosis, Are They Worth the Cancer Risk?" *Modern Medicine* 45, no. 9 (1977): 15.

Hargrove, T. Joel, et al. "Menopausal Hormone Replacement Therapy with Continuous Daily Oral Micronized Estradiol and Progesterone." *Obstetrics and Gynecology* 73, no. 4 (1989): 606–12.

Jick, S. S. et al. "Risk of Idiopathic Cerebral Haemorrhage in Women on Oral Contraceptives with Differing Progestagen Components." *Lancet* 354 (1999): 302–3.

Lee, John R. "Hormonal and Nutritional Aspects of Osteoporosis." *Health and Nutrition* 6, no. 7 (1991): 4.

Lee, John R. "Is Natural Progesterone the Missing Link in Osteoporosis Prevention and Treatment?" *Medical Hypotheses* 35 (1991): 316, 318.

Lee, John R. "Osteoporosis Reversal: The Role of Progesterone." *International Clinical Nutrition Review* 10, no. 3 (1990): 384–91.

Lee, John R. "Significance of Molecular Configuration Specificity—The Case of Progesterone and Osteoporosis." *Townsend Letter for Doctors*, (June 1993), 558.

Morter, M. T., Jr. "Osteoporosis!!" *The Chiropractic Professional*, May/June 1987.

Peat, Raymond F. *Progesterone in Orthomolecular Medicine*. Portland, Oreg.: Foundation for Hormonal and Nutrition Research, 1977.

Poulter, N. R., et al. "Effect on Stroke of Different Progestagens in Low Oestrogen Dose Oral Contraceptive." *Lancet* 254 (1999).

Prior, J. C. "Progesterone as a Bone-Trophic Hormone." *Endocrine Reviews* 11, no. 2 (1990): 386–98.

Prior, J. C., et al. "Progesterone and the Prevention of Osteoporosis." *Canadian Journal of OB/Gyn and Women's Health Care* 3, no. 4 (1991): 181.

Prior, J. C., et al. "Spinal Bone Loss and Ovulatory Disturbances." *International Journal of Gynecology and Obstetrics* 34 (1990): 253–56.

Riggs, B. L., et al. "Effect of Fluoride Treatment on Fracture Rate in Postmenopausal Women with Osteoporosis." *New England Journal of Medicine* 322 (1990): 802–9.

## Dietary Fats

Aylsworth, C. F., et al. "Effect of Fatty Acids on Junctional Communication: Possible Role in Tumor Promotion by Dietary Fat." *Lipids* 22, no. 6 (1987): 445–54.

Boutard, V., et al. "Fish Oil Supplementation and Essential Fatty Acid Deficiency Reduce Nitric Oxide Synthesis by Rat Macrophages." *Kidney International* 46, no. 5 (1994): 1280–86.

Chemla, D., et al. "Influence of Dietary Polyunsaturated Fatty Acids on Contractility, Inotropy and Compliance of Isolated Rate Myocardium." *Journal of Molecular and Cellular Cardiology* 27, no. 8, (1995): 1745–55.

Cleland, I. G., et al. "Clinical and Biochemical Effects of Dietary Fish Oil Supplements in Rheumatoid Arthritis." *Journal of Rheumatology* (1988).

Clinton, S. K., et al. "The Combined Effects of Dietary Fat and Estrogen on Survival. 7,12-Dimethyl-benz(a)-Anthracene-Induced Breast Cancer and Prolactin Metabolism in Rats." *Journal of Nutrition* 125, no. 5 (1995): 1192–1204.

Clouatre, Dallas. *Anti-Fat Nutrients.* San Francisco: Pax Publishing, 1995, 137.

Darmani, H., et al. "Interferon-Gamma and Polyunsaturated Fatty Acids Increase the Binding of Lipopolysaccharide to Macrophages." *International Journal of Experimental Pathology* 75, no. 5 (1994): 363–68.

Erasmus, Udo. *Fats That Heal. Fats That Kill.* Vancouver, B.C., Canada: Alive Books, 1997, 98.

Felton, C. V., et al. "Dietary Polyunsaturated Fatty Acids and Composition of Human Aortic Plaques." *Lancet* 334, no. 8931 (1994): 1195–96.

Geusens, C., et al. "Long-term Effect of Omega-3 Fatty Acid Supplementation in Active Rheumatoid Arthritis." *Arthritis and Rheumatism* 37 (1994): 824–29.

Henry, C. J., et al. "Protein Utilization, Growth and Survival in Essential Fatty-Acid-Deficient Rats." *British Journal of Nutrition* 75, no. 2 (1996): 237–48.

Houssay, B. A., and C. Martinez. "Experimental Diabetes and Diet." *Science* 105 (1947): 548–49.

Houssay, B. A., et al. "Accion de la administracion prolongada de glucosa sobre la diabetes de la rata." *Revista sociedad Argentina de biologia* 23 (1994): 288–93.

Imaizumi, K., et al. "Dissociation of Protein Kinase C. Activities and Diacylglycerol Levels in Liver Plasma Membranes of Rats on Coconut Oil and Safflower Oil Diets." *Journal of Nutritional Biochemistry* 6, no. 10 (1995): 528–33.

Kremer, J. M., et al. "Dietary Fish Oil and Olive Oil Supplementation in Patients with Rheumatoid Arthritis." *Arthritis and Rheumatism* 33, no. 6 (1990): 810–20.

Kremer, J. M., et al. "Effects of High Dose Fish Oil on Rheumatoid Arthritis After Stopping Nonsteroidal Antiinflammatory Drugs." *Arthritis and Rheumatism* 38 (1995): 1107–14.

Kremer, J. M., et al. "Fish-Oil Fatty Acid Supplementation in Active Rheumatoid Arthritis." *Annals of Internal Medicine* 106, no. 4 (1987): 497–503.

Kudryavtsev, I. A., et al. "Character of the Modifying Action of Polyunsaturated Fatty Acids on Growth of Transplantable Tumors of Various Types." *Bulletin of Experimental Biology and Medicine* 105, no. 4 (1986): 567–70.

Lucas, C., et al. "Dietary Fat Aggravates Active Rheumatoid Arthritis." *Clinical Research* 29, (abstract) no. 754A (1981).

Lynch, R. D. "Utilization of Polyunsaturated Fatty Acids by Human Diploid Cells Aging in Vitro." *Lipids* 15, no. 6 (1967): 412–20.

Mascioli, E. A., et al. "Unsaturated Fats Directly Kill White Blood Cells." *Lipids* 22, no. 6 (1987): 421.

Meade, C. J., and J. Martin. *Advances in Lipid Research* 127 (1978).

Olea, Sanchez, et al. "Inhibition by Polyunsaturated Fatty Acids of Cell Volume Regulation and Osmolyte Fluxes in Astrocytes." *American Journal of Physiology—Cell Physiology* 38, no. 1 (1995): C96–C102.

Pearce, M. L., and S. Dayton. "Incidence of Cancer in Men on a Diet High in Polyunsaturated Fat." *Lancet* 1 (1971): 464–67.

Pryor, W. A. "Free Radicals and Lipid Peroxidation—What They Are and How They Got That Way." *Natural Antioxidants in Humans* (1994): 1–24.

Purasiri, P., et al. "Modulation of Cytokine Production in Vivo by Dietary Essential Fatty Acids in Patients with Colorectal Cancer." *Clinical Science* 87, no. 6 (1994): 711–17.

Selye, Hans. "Sensitization by Corn Oil for the Production of Cardiac Necrosis." *American Journal of Cardiology* 23 (1969): 719–22.

Street, D. A., et al. "Serum Antioxidants and Myocardial Infarction—Are Low Levels of Carotenoids and Alph-tocopherol Risk Factors for Myocardial Infarction?" *Circulation* 90, no. 3 (1994): 1154–61.

Takei, M., et al. "Inhibitory Effects of Calcium Antagonists on Mitochondrial Swelling Induced by Lipid Peroxidation or Arachidonic Acid in the Rat Brain in Vitro." *Neurochemical Research* 29, no. 9 (1994): 1199–1206.

Tappia, P. S., et al. "Influence of Unsaturated Fatty Acids on the Production of Tumor Necrosis Factor and Interleukin-6 by Rat Peritoneal Macrophages." *Molecular and Cellular Biochemistry* 143, no. 2 (1995): 89–98.

## NutraSweet and Disease

Camfield, P. R., et al. "Aspartame Exacerbates EEG Spike-Wave Discharge in Children with Generalized Absence Epilepsy: A Double-Blind Controlled Study." *Neurology* 42 (1992): 1000–003.

Hicks, M. "NutraSweet . . . Too Good to Be True?" *General Aviation News*, 31 July 1989.

McCann, Joseph E. *Sweet Success: How NutraSweet Created a Billion Dollar Business*. Homewood, Ill: Business One Irwin, 1990.

Monte, W. C. "Aspartame: Methanol and the Public Health." *Journal of Applied Nutrition* 36 (1984): 41–52.

Remington, Dennis W. *The Bitter Truth About Artificial Sweeteners*. Provo, Utah: Vitality House International, 1987.

Roberts, H. *Aspartame (NutraSweet): Is It Safe?* Philadelphia: Charles Press, 1990.

Roberts, H. "Does Aspartame Cause Human Brain Cancer?" *Journal of Advancement in Medicine* 4, no. 4 (1991): 231–41.

Walton, R. D., et al. "Adverse Reactions to Aspartame: Double-blind Challenge in Patients from a Vulnerable Population." *Biological Psychiatry* 34 (1993): 13–17.

## Nerve Interference Ultimately Leading to Inflammation

Barnes, Tracy A. "Attention Deficit Hyperactivity Disorder and the Triad of Health." *Journal of Clinical Chiropractic Pediatrics* 1, no. 2 (1996): 59–65.

Brown, Mary, and Paul Vaillancourt. "Case Report: Upper Cervical Adjusting for Knee Pain." *Chiropractic Research Journal* 2, no. 4 (1993).

Bryner, P., and P. G. Staerker. "Indigestion and Heartburn: A Descriptive Study of Prevalence in Persons Seeking Care from Chiropractors." *Journal of Manipulative and Physiological Therapeutics* 19, no. 5 (1996): 317–23.

Cailliet, Rene. "Adhesive Capsulitis: The 'Frozen Shoulder.'" In *Shoulder Pain*. Philadelphia: F. A. Davis Co., 1982, 88.

Collins, Karen Feeley, and Bruce Pfleger. "The Neurophysiological Evaluation of the Subluxation Complex: Documenting the Neurological Component with Somatosensory Potentials." *Chiropractic Research Journal* 3, no. 1 (1994).

Cox, J. M., and S. Shreiner. "Chiropractic Manipulation in Low Back Pain and Sciatica; Statistic Data on the Diagnosis, Treatment and Response of 576 Consecutive Cases." *Journal of Manipulative and Physiological Therapeutics* 7, no. 1 (1984): 1–11.

Dabbs, V., and W. J. Lauretti. "A Risk Assessment of Cervical Manipulation vs. NSAIDs for the Treatment of Neck Pain." *Journal of Manipulative and Physiological Therapeutics* 18, no. 8 (1995): 530–36.

Daly, J. M., P. S. Frame, and P. A. Rapoza. "Sacroiliac Subluxation: A Common Treatable Cause of Low Back Pain in Pregnancy." *Family Practice Research Journal* 11, no. 2 (1991): 149–59.

Dommisse, G. F., and R. P. Grahe. "The Failure of Surgery for Lumbar Disc Disorders." *Disorder of the Lumbar Spine* (1978).

Dunn, E. E. "Osteopathic Concepts in Psychiatry." *Journal of the American Osteopathic Association* 49 (1950): 354–57.

Eriksen, Kirk. "Correction of Juvenile Idiopathic Scoliosis After Primary Upper Cervical Chiropractic Care: A Case Study." *Chiropractic Research Journal* 3, no. 3 (1996).

Eriksen, Kirk, and Edward F. Owens, Jr. "Upper Cervical Post X-Ray

Reduction and its Relationship to Symptomatic Improvement and Spinal Stability." *Chiropractic Research Journal* 4, no. 1 (1997).

Fernandez, Peter G. *I Yelled for Help . . . but You Didn't Listen.* The Winner's Circle, 1983.

Fidelibus, J. C. "An Overview of Neuroimmunomodulation and a Possible Correlation with Musculoskeletal System Function." *Journal of Manipulative and Physiological Therapeutics* 12, no. 4 (1989): 289–92.

Fredrick, H. E., et al. "The Chiropractic Vertebral Subluxation and Its Relationship to Vertebrogenic Lumbar Pain, Cruralgia and Sciatic Syndromes." *Chiropractic Research Journal* 3, no. 2 (1996).

Froehle, R. M. "Ear Infection: A Retrospective Study Examining Improvement from Chiropractic Care and Analyzing for Influencing Factors." *Journal of Manipulative and Physiological Therapeutics* 19, no. 3 (1996): 169–77.

Fuhr, A. W., and P. J. Osterbauer. "Interexaminer Reliability of Relative Leg Length Evaluations in the Prone Extended Position." *Chiropractic Technique* 1, no. 1 (1989): 13–18.

Giesen, J. M., et al. "An Evaluation of Chiropractic Manipulation as a Treatment of Hyperactivity in Children." *Journal of Manipulative and Physiological Therapeutics* 12 no. 5 (1989): 353–63.

Grostic, John D. "The Adjusting Instrument as a Research Tool." *Chiropractic Research Journal* 1, no. 2 (1988).

Herzberg, U., et al. "Spinal Cord NMDA Receptors Modulate Peripheral Immune Responses and Spinal Cord c-fos Expression After Immune Challenge in Rats Subjected to Unilateral Mononeuropathy." *Journal of Neuroscience* 16, no. 2 (1996): 730–43.

Hoiris, Kathryn T., et al. "Design and Implementation of a Randomized Controlled Trial of Chiropractic Care Versus Drug Therapy for Sub-Acute Low Back Pain." *Chiropractic Research Journal* 4, no. 2 (1997).

Hviid, C. "A Comparison of the Effects of Chiropractic Treatment on Respiratory Function in Patients with Respiratory Distress Symptoms and Patients without." *Bulletin of the European Chiropractic Union* 26 (1978): 17–34.

Keller, Tony S., et al. "Validation of the Force and Frequency Characteristics of the Activator Adjusting Instrument: Effectiveness as a Mechanical Impedance Measurement Tool." *Journal of Manipulative and Physiological Therapeutics* 22, no. 2 (1999): 75–86.

Killinger, L. "Chiropractic Care in the Treatment of Asthma." *Palmer Journal of Research* 2, no. 3 (1995): 74–77.

Knutson, Gary A. "Tonic Neck Reflexes, Leg Length Inequality and Atlanto-Occipital Fat Pad Impingement: An Atlas Subluxation Complex Hypothesis." *Chiropractic Research Journal* 4, no. 2 (1997).

Kokjohn, K., et al. "The Effect of Spinal Manipulation on Pain and Prostaglandin Levels in Women with Primary Dysmenorrhea." *Journal of Manipulative and Physiological Therapeutics* 15, (1992): 279–85.

Koren, Tedd. *Sciatica and Leg Pain*. Philadelphia: Koren Publications, 1989.

Kurvers, H. A., et al. "The Spinal Component to Skin Blood Flow Abnormalities in Reflex Sympathetic Dystrophy." *Archives of Neurology* 53, 1 (1996): 58–65.

Lanas A., et al. "Evidence of Aspirin Use in Both Upper and Lower Gastrointestinal Perforation." *Gastroenterology* 112 (1997): 683–89.

Mathews, J. A., et al. "Back Pain and Sciatica: Controlled Trials of Manipulation, Traction, Sclerosant and Epidural Injections." *British Journal of Rheumatology* 26 (1987): 416–23.

McKnight, M. E., and K. F. DeBoer, "Preliminary Study of Blood Pressure Changes in Normotensive Subjects Undergoing Chiropractic Care." *Journal of Manipulative and Physiological Therapeutics* 11, no. 4 (1988): 261–66.

McPartland, J. M., R. R. Brodeur, and R. C. Hallgren. "Chronic Neck Pain, Standing Balance, and Suboccipital Muscle Atrophy—A Pilot Study." *Journal of Manipulative and Physiological Therapeutics* 20, no. 1 (1997): 24–29.

Mechler, Frank. "Review of the Anatomy, Histology and Clinical Significance of the Vertebral Artery in Health and Disease." *Chiropractic Research Journal* 1, no. 1 (1988).

Nielsen, N., and B. Christianson. "Prognostic Factors in Bronchial Asthma in Chiropractic Practice." *Journal of the Australian Chiropractic Association* 18, no. 3 (1988): 85–87.

Nielsen, N. H., et al. "Chronic Asthma and Chiropractic Spinal Manipulation: A Randomized Clinical Trial." *Clinical and Experimental Allergy* 25, no. 1 (1995): 80–88.

Owens, Edward F., et al. "Changes in General Health Status During Upper Cervical Chiropractic Care: PBR Progress Report." *Chiropractic Research Journal* 5, no. 1 (1998).

Phillips, N. J. "Vertebral Subluxation and Otitis Media: A Case Study." *Chiropractic* 8, no. 2. (1992): 38–39.

Pikalov, A. A., and V. V. Kharin. "Use of Spinal Manipulative Therapy in the Treatment of Duodenal Ulcer: A Pilot Study." *Journal of Manipulative and Physiological Therapeutics* 17, no. 5 (1994): 310–13.

Polkinghorn, B. S. "Posterior Calcaneal Subluxation: An Important Consideration in Chiropractic Treatment of Plantar Fasciitis (Heel Spur Syndrome)." *Chiropractic Sports Medicine* 9, no. 2 (1995): 44–51.

Polkinghorn, B. S. and C. J. Colloca. "Treatment of Symptomatic Lumbar Disc Herniation Utilizing Activator Methods Chiropractic Technique." *Journal of Manipulative and Physiological Therapeutics* 21, no. 3 (April 1998): 187–96.

Richards, G. L., et al. "Low Force Chiropractic Care of Two Patients with Sciatic Neuropathy and Lumbar Disc Herniation." *American Journal of Chiropractic Medicine* 3, no. 1 (1990): 25–32.

Schwartz, H. S. "Preliminary Analysis of 350 Mental Patients' Records Treated by Chiropractors." *Journal of the National Chiropractic Association* (1949): 12–15.

Scotty, L. Kirby. "A Case Study: The Effects of Chiropractic on Multiple Sclerosis." *Chiropractic Research Journal* 3, no. 1 (1994).

Sheres, Brian M. "Chiropractic Efficacy Progress Report: Treatment of Spinal Neuralgia, Cephalgia, Vertigo and Related Peripheral Conditions." *Chiropractic Research Journal* 2, no. 3 (1993).

Strang, Virgil V. *Essential Principles of Chiropractic.* Davenport, Iowa: Palmer College of Chiropractic, 1985.

Turek, S. *Orthopaedics—Principles and Their Application.* Philadelphia: J. B. Lippincott Company, 1983.

van Breda, W. M., et al. "A Comparative Study of the Health Status of Children Raised Under the Health Care Models of Chiropractic and Allopathic Medicine." *Journal of Chiropractic Research* 5 (1989): 101–3.

Vannerson, J. F. "Sympathetic Vascular Malfunctions in Disease." *The Digest of Chiropractic Economics*, September/October 1977, 8.

Waddell, G. "Chronic Low-Back Pain, Psychologic Distress, and Illness Behavior." *Spine* 9, no. 2 (1984): 209–13.

Walton, E. V. "Chiropractic Effectiveness with Emotional, Learning and Behavioral Impairments." *International Review of Chiropractic* 29 (1975): 21–22.

Webster, Sarah K., and Medhat Alattar. "Literature Review: Mechanisms of

Physiological Responses to Adjustment." *Chiropractic Research Journal* 6, no. 1 (1998).

Weil, J., et al. "Prophylactic Aspirin and Risk of Peptic Ulcer Bleeding." *BMJ* 310, no. 6983 (1995): 827–30.

Yates, R. G., et al. "Effects of Chiropractic Treatment on Blood Pressure and Anxiety: A Randomized Controlled Trial." *Journal of Manipulative and Physiological Therapeutics* 11, no. 6. (1988): 484–88.

Youngquist, M. W., et al. "Interexaminer Reliability of an Isolation Test for the Presence of an Upper Cervical Isolation Subluxation." *Journal of Manipulative and Physiological Therapeutics* 12 (1989): 93–97.

## Accidents and Birthing Trauma Leading to Joint Disease

Batmanghelidj, F. *How to Deal Simply with Back Pain and Rheumatoid Joint Pain.* Falls Church, Va.: Global Health Solutions, 1992.

Huff, D. S. "Cytomegalovirus Inclusions in 401 Consecutive Autopsies in Infants 2 Weeks to 2 Years: A High Incidence in Patients with SIDS." Paper presented at the interim meeting of the Society for Pediatric Pathology, Dallas, October 1986.

Lantz, C. A. "Immobilization Degeneration and the Fixation Hypothesis of Chiropractic Subluxations." *Chiropractic Research Journal* 1 (1988): 21–46.

Maynard, Joseph E. *Healing Hands.* Woodstock, Ga.: Jonorm Publishing Company, 1991.

Molz, G., and H. Hartmann. Letter to the Editor. "Dysmorphism, Dysplasia and Anomaly in Sudden Infant Death." *New England Journal of Medicine* 311, no. 259 (1984).

Schneier, Monroe, et al. "Atlanto-Occipital Hypermobility in Sudden Infant Death Syndrome." *Today's Chiropractic* 19, no. 1 (1990).

Towbin, Abraham. "Latent Spinal Cord and Brain Stem Injury in Newborn Infants." (Towbin-Winsor Report.) *Developmental Medicine and Child Neurology* 11 (1969): 54–68.

Towbin, Abraham. "Spinal Injury Related to the Syndrome of Sudden Death ('Crib-Death') in Infants." *The American Journal of Clinical Pathology* 49, no. 4 (1968).

Valdez-Dapena, M. "A Pathologist's Perspective on Possible Mechanisms in SIDS." *Annals of the New York Academy of Sciences* 533 (1988): 31–36.

Webster, Larry L. "Chiropractic Care During Pregnancy." *International Chiropractic Pediatric Association* (1988).

## Benefits of Chelation Therapy

Brecher, Harold, and Arline Brecher. *Forty Something Forever. A Consumer's Guide to Chelation Therapy and Other Heart-Savers.* Troup, Tex.: Health Savers Press, 1992.

Casdorph, H. R. "EDTA Chelation Therapy II, Efficacy in Brain Disorders." *Journal of Holistic Medicine* 3, no. 2 (1981): 101–11.

Casdorph, H. R. "EDTA Chelation Therapy III, Treatment of Peripheral Arterial Occlusion, an Alternative to Amputation." *Journal of Holistic Medicine* 5, no. 1 (1983): 3–15.

Cranton, E. M., et al. "Free Radical Pathology in Age-Associated Diseases: Treatment with EDTA Chelation, Nutrition, and Antioxidants." *Journal of Holistic Medicine* 6, no. 1 (1984): 6–37.

Hutton, M., et al. "The Quantities of Cadmium, Lead, Mercury and Arsenic Entering the U.K. Environment from Human Activities." *Science of the Total Environment* 57 (1986): 129–50.

Lanza, F., et al. "Differential Effects of Extra- and Intracellular Calcium Chelation on Human Platelet Function and Glycoprotein IIb-IIIa Complex Stability." *Nouvelle Revue Francaise d'Hematologie* 34, no. 1 (1992): 123–31.

Lin, J. L., et al. "Disappearance of Immune Deposits with EDTA Chelation Therapy in a Case of IGa Nephropathy." *American Journal of Nephrology* 12, no. 6 (1992): 457–60.

Olszewer, E., et al. "EDTA Chelation Therapy in Chronic Degenerative Disease." *Medical Hypotheses* 1 (1988): 41–49.

Sehnert, K. W., et al. "The Improvement in Renal Function Following EDTA Chelation and Multi-Vitamin Trace-Mineral Therapy: A Study in Creatinine Clearance." *Medical Hypotheses* 15, no. 3 (1984): 301–4.

Van Rij, A. M., et al. "Chelation Therapy for Intermittent Claudication. A Double-Blind, Randomized, Controlled Trial." *Circulation* 90, no. 3 (1994): 1194–99.

# Notes

## Introduction

1.  M. H. Weisman et al., "Measures of Bone Loss in Rheumatoid Arthritis," *Archives of Internal Medicine* 146, no. 4 (1986): 701–04, quoted in Jeffrey S. Bland, *The Inflammatory Disorders* (Gig Harbor, Wash.: Healthcomm, Inc., 1997), 276–97.

2.  Raymond Peat, *PMS to Menopause* (Eugene, Oreg.: International University, 1997), 21, 23, 45. See also B. B. Gerstman et al., "Oral Contraceptive Estrogen Dose and the Risk of Deep Venous Thromboembolic Disease," *American Journal of Epidemiology* 113 (1991): 32–36; B. V. Stadel, "Oral Contraceptives and Cardiovascular Disease," *New England Journal of Medicine* 305 (1981): 612; M. P. Vessey et al., "Investigation of Relation Between Use of Oral Contraceptives and Thromboembolic Disease," *British Medical Journal* 2 (1968): 199–205; and P. W. F. Wilson et al., "Postmenopausal Estrogen Use, Cigarette Smoking, and Cardiovascular Morbidity in Women over 50," *New England Journal of Medicine* 313, no. 17 (1985): 1038–43.

3.  Robert Atkins, "The Red Vitamin's Full Palette of Power," *Dr. Robert Atkins' Health Revelations* IV, no. 3 (March 1996): 3.

4.  Paavo O. Airola, *There Is A Cure for Arthritis* (West Nyack, N.Y.: Parker Publishing Company, 1968), xii.

5.  Raquel Martin, *Today's Health Alternative* (Tehachapi, Calif.: America West Publishers, 1992), 48.

## Chapter One

1.  Jason Theodosakis, Brenda Adderly, and Barry Fox, *The Arthritis Cure* (New York: St. Martin's Press, 1997), 2.

2.  T. Moore, "Prescription Drugs: Danger Within the Cure," *Los Angeles Times*, 4 April 1998, quoted in Ronald Lawrence, "Inflammatory Drugs for Aching Joints Could Send You to the Hospital," *Journal of Longevity* 4, no. 6 (1998): 21.

3.  Stuart M. Berger, *How to be Your Own Nutritionist* (New York: William Morrow and Company, 1987), 173.

4.  B. Kowsari et al., "Assessment of the Diet of Patients with Rheumatoid Arthritis and Osteoarthritis," *Journal of the American Dietetic Association* 82, no. 6 (1983): 657–59. See also J. Kremer and J. Bigdouette, "Nutrient Intake of Patients with Rheumatoid Arthritis Is Deficient in Pyroxidine, Zinc, Copper and Magnesium," *Journal of Rheumatology* 23, no. 6 (1996): 990–94; E. C. Barton-Wright et al., "The Pantothenic Acid Metabolism of Rheumatoid Arthritis," *Lancet* (1963): 862; and T. McAlindon et al., "Relation of Dietary Intake and Serum Levels of Vitamin D to Progression of Osteoarthritis of the Knee," *Annals of Internal Medicine* 125, no. 5 (1996): 353–59.

5.  Craig Weatherby and Leonid Gordin, *The Arthritis Bible* (Rochester, Vt.: Healing Arts Press, 1999), 59.

6.  Patricia Andersen-Parrado, "Homeopathic Remedies to Ease Acute and Chronic Arthritis Pain," *Better Nutrition*, February 1997, 26.

7.  Alex Duarte, *Jaws for Life: The Story of Shark Cartilage* (author, 1993) 9; see also Jane Heimlich, *What Your Doctor Won't Tell You* (New York: HarperCollins, 1990), 234; Julian Whitaker, "Clear Up Inflammation with Enzymes," *Dr. Julian Whitaker's Health and Healing* 8, no. 8 (August 1998): 1; and Geoffrey Cowley and Anne Underwood, "What Is SAMe?" *Newsweek*, 5 July 1999.

8.  J. Lazarou et al., "Incidence of Adverse Drug Reactions in Hospitalized Patients," *Journal of the American Medical Association* 279 (1998): 1200–1205.

9.  John R. Lee, *What Your Doctor May Not Tell You About Menopause* (New York: Warner Books, 1996), 257.

10. T. V. Perneger et al., "Risk of Kidney Failure Associated with the Use of Acetaminophen, Aspirin, and Nonsteroidal Anti-Inflammatory Drugs," *New England Journal of Medicine* 331, no. 25 (1994): 1675–79. See also and N. M. Newman et al., "Acetabular Bone Destruction Related to Nonsteroidal Anti-Inflammatory Drugs," *Lancet* 2, (1985): 11–14; and *Scandinavian Journal of Rheumatology* 91 (1991): 9–17, cited in Julian Whitaker, "NSAIDs Cause GI Bleeding and Cartilage Destruction," *Dr. Julian Whitaker's Health and Healing* 8, no. 5 (May 1998): 6.

11. Lazarou et al., "Incidence of Adverse Drug Reactions," 1200–1205.

12. D. L. Scott et al., "Long-term Outcome of Treating Rheumatoid Arthritis: Results After 20 Years," *Lancet* (1987).

13. Lawrence, "Inflammatory Drugs for Aching Joints," 21. See also Moore, "Prescription Drugs."

14. Trien Susan Falmholtz, *Change of Life* (New York: Fawcett Columbine Books, 1986).

15. L. V. Avioli, "Therapy Induced Osteoporosis," in *Osteoporosis: Physiological Basis, Assessment and Treatment* (New York: Elsevier, 1990).

16. James F. Balch and Phyllis A. Balch, *Prescription for Nutritional Healing* (Garden City Park, N.Y.: Avery Publishing Group, 1997), 336.

17. Robert S. Mendelsohn, "The People's Doctor," *Let's Live*, May 1987, 62.

18. William Boyd, *Textbook of Pathology*, 8th ed. (Philadelphia: Lea and Febiger, 1970), 18.

19. Heimlich, *What Your Doctor Won't Tell You*, 135.

20. Dr. William B. Rawls, "An Evaluation of the Present-Day Therapy in Rheumatoid Arthritis," *New York Medicine* (August 1947).

21. Airola, *There Is a Cure for Arthritis*, 39.

22. Ibid., 26.

23. Jeffrey S. Bland, *The Inflammatory Disorders* (Gig Harbor, Wash.: HealthComm, 1997), 11; and H. K. Liang, "Clinical Evaluation of the Poisoned Patient and Toxic Syndromes," *Clinical Chemistry* 42, no. 8B (1996): 1350–55.

24. Theodosakis, Adderly, and Fox, *The Arthritis Cure*, 154.

25. Julian Whitaker, "Clear Up Inflammation with Enzymes," 2.

26. Joe Graedon, *The People's Pharmacy* (New York: Avon Books, 1977), 2, 4, 19, 23, 24, 47.

27. Stanley Burroughs, *The Master Cleanser* (Auburn, Calif.: Burroughs Books, 1993), 8.

28. Airola, *There Is a Cure for Arthritis*, 174.

29. Burroughs, *The Master Cleanser*, 6.

30. Whitaker, "Clear Up Inflammation with Enzymes," 1–4.

31. Theodosakis, Adderly, and Fox, *The Arthritis Cure*, 162.

32. Bland, *The Inflammatory Disorders*, 298–307.

33. J. Prudden et al., "The Biological Activity of Bovine Cartilage Preparations," *Seminars in Arthritis and Rheumatism* 3, no. 4 (1974): 287.

34. Duarte, *Jaws for Life*, 31.

35. Atkins, *Dr. Robert Atkins' Health Revelations*, 5–6.

36. Ibid., 5.

37. J. Z. Miller et al., "Calcium Absorption from Calcium Carbonate and a New Form of Calcium (CCM) in Healthy Male and Female Adolescents," *American Journal of Clinical Nutrition* 48 (1988): 1291–94.

38. Raquel Martin and Judi Gerstung, *The Estrogen Alternative: Natural*

*Hormone Therapy with Botanical Progesterone*, 3rd ed. (Rochester, Vt.: Healing Arts Press, 1997), 121.

39.  A. C. Goyton and J. E. Hall, *Textbook of Medical Physiology* (Philadelphia: Saunders, 1996), 989.

40.  J. J. Stepan et al., "Prospective Trial of Ossein-Hydroxyapatite Compound in Surgically Induced Postmenopausal Women," *Bone* 10 (1989): 179–87.

41.  Beth M. Ley, *How to Fight Osteoporosis and Win* (Aliso Viejo, Calif.: BL Publications, 1996), 51–55.

42.  For information on minerals, see K. H. Nilsen, M. I. V. Jayson, and A. S. J. Dixon, "Microcrystalline Calcium Hydroxyapatite Compound in Corticosteroid-Treated Rheumatoid Patients: A Controlled Study," *British Medical Journal* 2 (October 1978): 1124. For information on vitamins, see Julian Whitaker, *147 Medically-Proven Miracle Cures*, (Potomac, Md.: Phillips Publishing, 1996), 7. Magnesium, manganese, phosphorus, zinc, copper, boron, nickel, rubidium, platinum, strontium, barium, potassium, and silica are some of the ingredients needed in the formation of bone. See Ley, *How to Fight Osteoporosis*, 54, 62. Vitamins C, D, $B_1$, and K are also present in mycrocrystalline hydroxyapatite. See James F. Scheer, "Osteoporosis: Calcium Is Just the Beginning," *Health Freedom News* 17, no. 3 (1998): 14.

43.  Nilsen, Jayson, and Dixon, "Microcrystalline Calcium Hydroxyapatite Compound," 1124.

44.  H. Siemandi, "The Effect of Cis-9-cetyl Myristoleate (CMO) and Adjunctive Therapy on Arthritis and Auto-Immune Disease: A Randomized Trial," *Townsend Newsletter for Doctors and Patients* 169 (August 1997): 58–63.

45.  Marcia Zimmerman, "Cetyl-Myristoleate," *Nature's Impact*, August/September 1998, 31–32.

46.  Morton Walker, "CM for Arthritis Sufferers," *Nutritional Medicine*, June 1998, 40.

47.  Kenneth Absher, "Harvard Scientists Find Nutrient Critical to Joint Problems," *Journal of Longevity* 4, no. 8 (1998): 13.

48.  Siemandi, "The Effect of Cis-9-Cetyl Myristoleate (CMO); H. Siemandi, "Cetyl Myristoleate—A Unique Natural Compound Valuable in Arthritis Conditions," 58–63.

49.  Zimmerman, "Cetyl-Myristoleate," 31–33.

50.  Theodosakis, Adderly, and Fox, *The Arthritis Cure*, 172.

51.  Lawrence, "Inflammatory Drugs for Aching Joints," *Journal of Longevity* 4, no. 6 (1998): 22. See also A. Conte, "Biochemical and

Pharmacokinetic Aspect of Oral Treatment with Chondroitin Sulfate," *Drug Research* 45, no. 8 (1995): 918–25.

52. Theodosakis, Adderly, and Fox, *The Arthritis Cure*, 42, 44.

53. Patricia Clarke, "Bone/Joint Problems—Can You Expect More Than Relief?" *Journal of Longevity* 5, no. 8 (1999): 19.

54. Kenneth Absher, "Harvard Scientists Find Nutrient Critical to Joint Problems," *Journal of Longevity* 4, no. 8 (1998): 12.

55. M. Barnett et al., "A Pilot Trial of Oral Type II Collagen in the Treatment of Juvenile Rheumatoid Arthritis," *Arthritis and Rheumatism* 39, no. 4 (1996): 623–28.

56. M. Barnett et al., "Treatment of Rheumatoid Arthritis with Oral Type II Collagen: Results of a Multicenter, Double-Blind, Placebo-Controlled Trial," *Arthritis and Rheumatism* 41, no. 2 (1998): 290–97. See also D. E. Trentham et al., "Effects of Oral Administration of Type II Collagen on Rheumatoid Arthritis," *Science* 261, no. 5129 (1993): 1727–30; D. Trentham et al., "Evidence That Type II Collagen Feeding Can Induce a Durable Therapeutic Response in Some Patients with Rheumatoid Arthritis," *Annals of the New York Academy of Sciences* 778 (1996): 306–14; and T. Geiger et al., "Effect on Collagen Induced Arthritis in DBA/l Mice," *Journal of Rheumatology* 21 (1994): 1992–97.

57. Barnett et al., "Treatment of Rheumatoid Arthritis," 290–97.

58. For information on joints, see J. Pujalte et al., "Double-Blind Clinical Evaluation of Oral Glucosamine Sulphate in the Basic Treatment of Osteoarthritis," *Current Medical Research and Opinion* 7, no. 2 (1980): 110–14; E. D'Ambrosio et al., "Glucosamine Sulfate: A Controlled Clinical Investigation of Arthrosis," *Pharmatherapeutica* 2, no. 8 (1981): 504; and M. Tapadinhas et al., "Oral Glucosamine Sulphate in the Management of Arthrosis: Report on a Multicentre Open Investigation in Portugal," *Pharmatherapeutica* 3, no. 3 (1982): 147–68.

59. Absher, "Harvard Scientists Find Nutrient Critical," 13.

60. For information on wound healing, see J. Prudden et al., "Bovine Cartilage Preparations," 287. "The Colostrum Miracle—Too Good to Be True?" *Vital Health News*, Winter 1998, 11.

61. Ibid., 6.

62. Lance Wright, "Suffering from an Autoimmune Disease?" *Alternative Medicine*, September 1999, 45.

63. S. M. Seyedin et al., "Cartilage Inducing Factor A; Apparent Identity to Transforming Growth Factor Beta," *Journal of Biological Chemistry* 261, no. 13 (1986): 5693–95.

64. Steve Schwade, "Insulin-like Growth Factor," *Muscle and Fitness* (May 1992): 80–81.

65. Prudden et al., "The Colostrum Miracle," 5.

66. Wright, "Suffering from an Autoimmune Disease?" 45.

67. Daniel G. Clark and Kaye Wyatt, *Colostrum* (Salt Lake City, Utah: CNR Publications, 1996), 69.

68. J. M. Dwyer, "Manipulating the Immune System with Immune Globulin," *New England Journal of Medicine* 326, no. 2 (1992): 107.

69. *Physician's Desk Reference: Consumer's Guide to Nonprescription Drugs* (Oradell, N.J.: Medical Economics, 1987), 772.

70. Jane Heimlich, *What Your Doctor Won't Tell You,* (New York: HarperCollins Publishers, 1990), 156.

71. John R. J. Sorenson, "Copper Chelates as Possible Active Metabolites of the Antiarthritic and Antiepileptic Drugs," *Journal of Applied Nutrition* 32, no. 1 (1980): 4–25, cited in Heimlich, *What Your Doctor Won't Tell You.*

72. Julian M. Whitaker, *99 Secrets for a Longer Healthier Life* (Potomac, Md.: Phillips Publishing, 1992), 17–18.

73. Julian Whitaker, "DMSO Protects the Spine in Acute Phase," *Dr. Julian Whitaker's Health and Healing* (supplement) (May 1998): 1–2.

74. J. C. Coles et al., "Role of Free Radical Scavenger in Protection of Spinal Cord During Ischemia," *Annals of Thoracic Surgery* 41 (1986): 551–56.

75. Pat McGrady, *The Persecuted Drug—The Story of DMSO,* rev. ed. (New York: Charter Books, 1979), 274.

76. Ibid., vii.

77. Julian Whitaker, "Why DMSO Is Such a Remarkable Therapeutic Agent," *Dr. Julian Whitaker's Health and Healing* 5, no. 8 (1995): 2, 3.

78. David Williams, "Dangers of Alternative Medicine," *The Worldwide Journal of Lifelong Health,* Fall 1998, 22.

79. McGrady, *The Persecuted Drug,* 95.

80. For information on reducing pain in joints, see Theodosakis, Adderly, and Fox, *The Arthritis Cure,* 11, 13; and A. Drovanti et al., "Therapeutic Activity of Oral Glucosamine Sulfate in Osteoarthritis: A Placebo Double-Blind Investigation," *Clinical Therapeutics,* 3 (1980): 260. For information on side effects, see *Exercise and Your Arthritis* (Atlanta: The Arthritis Foundation, January 1996), brochure no. 835-54555; and Pujalte et al., "Double-Blind Clinical Evaluation," 114.

81. M. J. Tapadinhas et al., "Oral Glucosamine Sulphate in the Management of Arthrosis: Report on a Multi-Centre Open Investigation in Portugal," *Pharmatherapeutica* 3, no. 3 (1982): 157–68; and Pujalte et al., "Double-Blind Clinical Evaluation," 110–114.

82. I. Setnikar et al., "Antiarthritic Effects of Glucosamine Sulfate Studies in Animal Models," *Arzmeo-Forsch/Drug Research* 41, no. 1 (1991): 542–45.

83. D'Ambrosio et al., "Glucosamine Sulphate," 504–8.

84. Pujalte et al., "Double-Blind Clinical Evaluation," 110–14.

85. Al Vaz, "Double Blind Clinical Evaluation of the Relative Efficacy of Ibuprofen and Glucosamine Sulfate in the Management of Osteoarthritis of the Knee in Out-patients," *Current Medical Research and Opinion* 8 (1982): 145–49.

86. Michael T. Murray, "Irrefutable Evidence: Glucosamine Sulfate Proven Superior Over Other Forms of Glucosamine and Chondroitin Sulfate," *Vital Communications* (brochure), 30 May 1997.

87. For information on low levels of glucosamine in arthritis patients, see M. X. Sullivan et al., "Cystine Content of Finger Nails in Arthritis," *Journal of Bone and Joint Surgery* 16 (1935): 185–88; and B. D. Senturia, "Results of Treatment of Chronic Arthritis and Rheumatoid Conditions with Colloidal Sulphur," *Journal of Bone and Joint Surgery* 16 (1934): 119–25. For information on the benefits of supplementation, see Tapadinhas et al., "Oral Glucosamine Sulfate," 157–68.

88. Doss, "Bone Health," 12; and G. Crolle et al., "Glucosamine Sulfate for the Management of Arthrosis: A Controlled Clinical Investigation," *Current Medical Research and Opinion* 7 (1980): 104–9.

89. Theodosakis, Adderly, and Fox, *The Arthritis Cure*. See 44 for the first quote, 47 for the second quote, and 55 for information on dosages.

90. R. W. Hong et al., "Glutamine Protects the Liver Following Corynebacterium Parvum/Endotoxin-Induced Hepatic Necrosis," *Surgical Forum* 42 (1991): 1–3.

91. John R. Lee, "Interview with Marc Rose, M.D.," *The John R. Lee, M.D. Medical Letter* (June 1999): 6.

92. A. Bruce et al., "The Effect of Selenium and Vitamin E on Glutathione Peroxidase Levels and Subjective Symptoms in Patient with Arthrosis and Rheumatoid Arthritis," in *Proceedings of the New Zealand Workshop on Trace Elements in New Zealand* (Otago, New Zealand: Dundin University of Otago, 1981), 92, cited in Weatherby and Gordin, *The Arthritis Bible*, 124.

93. Judy Shabert et al., *The Ultimate Nutrient Glutamine: The Essential Nonessential Amino Acid* (Garden City Park, N.Y.: Avery Publishing Group, 1994), 62–63.

94. Jack Challem, *The Nutrition Reporter* 8, no. 7 (July 1997).

95. S. Adami et al., "Ipriflavone Prevents Radial Bone Loss in Postmeno-pausal Women with Low Bone Mass Over 2 Years," *Osteoporosis International* 7 (1997): 23–28. See also D. Agnusdei et al., "A Double-Blind, Placebo-Controlled Trial of Ipriflavone for Prevention of Post-Menopausal Bone Loss," *Calcified Tissue International* 61 (1997): 141–47; and M. Passeri et al., "Effects of 2-Year Therapy with Ipriflavone in Elderly Women with Established Osteoporosis," *Italian Journal of Mineral and Electrolyte Metabolism* 9 (1995): 137–44.

96. Anthony L. Almada, "Ipriflavone: The New Bone Builder," *Nutrition Science News* 3, no. 4 (1998): 198. See also K. Notoya et al., "Inhibitory Effect of Ipriflavone on Osteoclast-Mediated Bone Resorption and New Osteoclast Formation in Long-term Cultures of Mouse Unfractionated Bone Cells," *Calcified Tissue International* 53, no. 3 (1993): 206–9; S. Benvenuti et al., "Binding and Bioeffects of Ipriflavone on a Human Preosteoclastic Line," *Biochemical and Biophysical Research Communications* 201, no. 3 (1994): 1084–89; and A. Myauchi et al., "Novel Ipriflavone Receptors Coupled to Calcium Influx Regulate Osteoclast Differentiation and Function," *Endocrinology* 13, no. 8 (1996): 3544–50.

97. A. Barbul, "Arginine: Biochemistry, Physiology and Therapeutic Implications," *Journal of Parenteral and Enteral Nutrition* 10 (1986): 227–38.

98. Elisabeth-Anne Cole, "The Silent Threat to Men and Women," *Journal of Longevity Research* 3, no. 6 (1997): 30.

99. R. Civitelli et al., "Dietary L-Lysine and Calcium Metabolism in Humans," *Nutrition* 8 (1992): 400–05.

100. Joe M. Elrod, *Reversing Fibromyalgia* (Pleasant Grove, Utah: Wood-land Publishing, 1997), 23.

101. *Journal of Rheumatology* 22, no. 5 (1995): 953–58.

102. B. M. Altura et al., "Magnesium and Cardiovascular Biology: An Important Link Between Cardiovascular Risk Factors and Atherogenesis," *Cellular and Molecular Biology Research* 4, no. 5 (1995): 347–59.

103. S. Weintraub, *Natural Treatments for ADD and Hyperactivity* (Pleasant Grove, Utah: Woodland Publishing, 1997).

104. Clarke, "Bone/Joint Problems," 20.

105. R. Lawrence, "Methylsulfonylmethane (M.S.M.): A Double-Blind Study of Its Use in Degenerative Arthritis," *International Journal of Anti-Aging Medicine* 1, no. 1 (1998): 50. See also B. Ley, *On Our Way Back with Sulfur* (Aliso Viejo, Calif.: BL Publications, 1998).

106. S. Jacob et al., *The Miracle of MSM: The Natural Solution for Pain* (New

York: Putnam, 1999); and M. Christy, *MSM, The Super-Supplement of the Decade* (Scottsdale, Ariz.: Wishland Publishing, 1997).

107. Earl L. Mindell, *The MSM Miracle* (New Canaan, Conn.: Keats Publishing, 1997), 10–12.

108. Ibid., 12.

109. Ibid., 12.

110. Ibid., 40.

111. Bob Delmoneque, "Critical Factor Discovered for Bone/Joint Repair," *Journal of Longevity* 5, no. 6 (1999).

112. Mindell, *The MSM Miracle*, 40.

113. Ibid., 41.

114. Stanley Jacob, "Preliminary Evaluation of MSM in Osteoarthritis," Oregon Health Sciences University, Portland (April 1997).

115. Linda G. Rector-Page, *Healthy Healing: An Alternative Healing* (Carmel Valley, Calif.: Healthy Healing Publications, 1992), 91.

116. A. Pfister et al., "Fixation Sites of Procyanidolic Oligomers in the Blood Capillary Walls of Lungs of Guinea Pigs," *Acta Physiologica Pharmacologica et Therapeutica Latinoamericana* (1982): 8, cited in Bert Schwitters et al., *OPC in Practice* (Rome: Alfa Omega Editrice, 1993), 58. See also J. Masquelier et al., *Acta Physiologica Pharmacologica et Therapeutica Latinoamericana* 7 (1981): 101–5, cited in Schwitters et al., *OPC in Practice*, 148; R. Kuttan et al., "Collagen Treated with (+) Catechin Becomes Resistant to the Action of Mammalian Collagenases," *Experientia* 37, no. 3 (1981): 2221–23; and J. M. Tixier et al., "Evidence by in Vivo and in Vitro Studies that Binding of Pycnogenols to Elastin Affects its Rate of Degradation by Elastases," *Biochemical Pharmacology* 33, no. 24 (1984): 3933–39.

117. Weatherby and Gordin, *The Arthritis Bible*, 157.

118. Rector-Page, *Healthy Healing: An Alternative Reference*, 69.

119. Robert D. Willix, Jr., *Health and Longevity* 2, no. 1 (January 1995).

120. Rita Elkins, *SAMe* (Pleasant Grove, Utah: Woodland Publishing, 1999), 6.

121. Sol Grazi, *SAMe (S-adenosylmethionine)* (Rocklin, Calif.: Prima Publishing, 1999), 93.

122. Elkins, *SAMe*, 24–25.

123. Elkins, *SAMe*, 6.

124. Grazi, *SAMe (S-adenosylmethionine)*, quotes on 89 and 156, respectively.

125. G. Stramentinoli, "Pharmacologic Aspects of S-adenosylmethionine,

Pharmacokinetics and Pharmacodynamics," *American Journal of Medicine* 83, no. 5A (1987): 35–42. See also M. F. Harmand et al., "Effects of S-Adenosylmethionine on Human Articular Chondrocyte Differentiation. An In Vitro Study," *American Journal of Medicine* 83, no. 5A (1987): 48–54; and C. di Padova, "S-Adenosylmethionine in the Treatment of Osteoarthritis. Review of the Clinical Studies," *American Journal of Medicine* 83, no. 5A (1987): 60–65; all three cited in Weatherby and Gordin, *The Arthritis Bible*, 47.

126. Elkins, *SAMe*, 6; and Cowley and Underwood, "What Is SAMe?"

127. Grazi, *SAMe (S-adenosylmethionine)*, 48.

128. O. Sanchez Pernaute et al., "SAMe Restores the Changes in the Proliferation and in the Synthesis of Fibroxectin and Proteoglycans Induced by Tumor Necrosis Factor Alpha on Cultured Rabbit Synovial Cells," *British Journal of Rheumatology* 36, no. 1 (1997): 27–31; and B. Konig, "A Long-term Clinical Trial with S-adenosylmethionine for the Treatment of Osteoarthritis," *American Journal of Medicine* 83, no. 5A (1987): 89–94.

129. P. DiBenedetto et al., "Clinical Evaluation of S-adenosylmethionine Versus Transcutaneous Electrical Nerve Stimulation in Primary Fibromyalgia," *Current Therapeutic Research* 53, no. 2 (1993): 222. See also H. Tavoni et al., "Evaluation of S-adenosylmethionine in Primary Fibromyalgia: A Double-Blind Crossover Study," *American Journal of Medicine* 83, no. 5A (1987): 107–10; S. Jacobsen et al., "Oral SAMe and Primary Fibromyalgia," *Scandinavian Journal of Rheumatology* 20, no. 4 (1991): 294–302; and A. Ianniello et al., "S-adenosylmethionine in Sjögren's Syndrome and Fibromyalgia," *Current Therapeutic Research* 55, no. 6 (1994): 699–706.

130. Grazi, *SAMe (S-adenosylmethionine)*. For information on the liver, see 145. For information on depression, see 28.

131. Grazi, *SAMe (S-adenosylmethionine)*, 216–17.

132. Elkins, *SAMe*, 24–25.

133. Duarte, *Jaws for Life*, 10, 12.

134. Ibid.; and A. J. Bollet, "Stimulation of Protein-Chondroitin Synthesis by Normal and Osteo Arthritic Articular Cartilage," *Arthritis and Rheumatism* 11 (1968): 663.

135. I. William Lane and Linda Comac, *Sharks Don't Get Cancer* (Garden City Park, N.Y.: Avery Publishing Group, 1992), 12.

136. Ibid, 118, 131.

137. Atkins, *Dr. Robert Atkins' Health Revelations*, 6.

138. Duarte, *Jaws for Life*, 10, 12.

139. Klaus Kaufmann, *Silica: The Amazing Gel* (Vancouver, B.C., Canada: Alive Books, 1992), 136.

140. Ibid., 3, 4.

141. Whitaker, *147 Medically-Proven Miracle Cures*, 7.

142. Rector-Page, *Healthy Healing: An Alternative Reference*, 69.

143. James F. Balch and Phyllis Balch, *Prescription for Nutritional Healing* (Garden City Park, N.Y.: Avery Publishing Group, 1997), 21.

144. Stephen T. Sinatra, *Optimum Health* (New York: The Lincoln-Bradley Publishing Group, 1996), 210.

145. Gaby, *Preventing and Reversing Osteoporosis*, 80. See also N. R. Calhoun et al., "The Effects of Zinc on Ectopic Bone Formation," *Oral Surgery* 39 (1975): 698–706.

146. T. McAlindon et al., "Relation of Dietary Intake and Serum Levels of Vitamin D to Progression of Osteoarthritis of the Knee," *Annals of Internal Medicine* 125, no. 5 (1996): 648–56, cited in Weatherby and Gordin, *The Arthritis Bible*, 125; P. A. Simkin, "Treatment of Rheumatoid Arthritis with Oral Zinc Sulfate," *Agents and Actions* (supplements) 8 (1981): 8578–95; P. C. Mattingly et al., "Zinc Sulphate in Rheumatoid Arthritis," *Annals of the Rheumatic Diseases* 41 (1982): 456–57; and S. P. Pandley et al., "Zinc in Rheumatoid Arthritis," *Indian Journal Medical Research* 81 (1985): 618–20.

147. Morton Walker, *The Chelation Way* (Garden City Park, N.Y.: Avery Publishing Group, 1990).

148. Walker, *The Chelation Way*, 55.

149. Scheer, "Osteoporosis: Calcium Is Just the Beginning," 14.

150. Rector-Page, *Healthy Healing*, ninth ed. (1994), 19.

151. Yves Requen, *Chi Kung: The Chinese Art of Mastering Energy* (Rochester, Vt.: Inner Traditions, 1995).

152. Dr. Harvey Green, "Fit for America: Health, Fitness, Sport, and American Society 1830–1940," televised interview, cited in Jack Soltanoff, *Natural Healing* (New York: Warner Books, 1988), 5.

153. Dava Sobel and Arthur C. Klein, *Arthritis: What Exercises Work* (New York: St. Martin's Press, 1995), 57–60.

154. F. Batmanghelidj, *Your Body's Many Cries for Water*, (Falls Church, Va.: Global Health Solutions, 1992), 15.

155. Batmanghelidj, *Your Body's Many Cries for Water*, quotes on 43 and 45, respectively.

156. Paul C. Bragg, *Water: The Shocking Truth That Can Save Your Life* (Calif.: Health Science), quoted in George H. Malkmus, *God's Way to Ultimate Health* (Eidson, Tenn.: Hallelujah Acres Publishing, 1997), 175.

157. Malkmus, *God's Way to Ultimate Health*, 178.

158. Norman W. Walker, *Water Can Undermine Your Health* (Prescott, Ariz.: Norwalk Press, 1974).

159. Malkmus, *God's Way to Ultimate Health*, 174.

160. Ibid., 182. For information on the positive effects of the distillation process, see 173, 175, 182.

161. F. Batmanghelidj, *How to Deal with Back Pain and Rheumatoid Joint Pain* (Falls Church, Va.: Global Health Solutions, 1991), 52. See also A. D. Cicoria and H. G. Hempling, "Osmotic Properties of Differentiating Bone Marrow Precursor Cells: Membrane Permeability to Non-Electrolytes," *Journal of Cellular Physiology* 105 (1980): 129–36.

162. Batmanghelidj, *How to Deal with Back Pain*, 56.

163. Ibid., 53.

164. F. Batmanghelidj, "Pain: A Need for Paradigm Change," *Anticancer Research* 7, no. 5B (1987): 971–90.

165. Batmanghelidj, *How to Deal with Back Pain*, 68. See also P. A. Phillips et al., "Reduced Thirst after Deprivation in Healthy Elderly Men," *New England Journal of Medicine* 311, no. 12 (1984): 753–59; Editorial, "Thirst and Osmoregulation in the Elderly," *Lancet* 2, no. 841 (1984): 1017–18; and B. Streen et al., "Body Water in the Elderly," *Lancet* (1985): 101.

166. Batmanghelidj, *How to Deal with Back Pain*, viii. See also E. Katchalski-Katzier, "Conformational Change in Macromolecules," *Biorheology* 21 (1984): 57–74.

## Chapter Two

1. Kurt W. Donsbach, *Arthritis* (Rosarito Beach, Baja, Calif.: Wholistic Publications, 1981), 3.

2. Ibid.

3. Paavo O. Airola, *There Is a Cure for Arthritis* (West Nyack, N.Y.: Parker Publishing, 1968), 30; Humbart Santillo, *Food Enzymes—The Missing Link to Radiant Health* (Prescott, Ariz.: Holm Press, 1987), 9.

4. Airola, *There Is a Cure for Arthritis*, 31, 154.

5. Julian Whitaker, "The FDA Blocks Health Claims That Can Help You," *Dr. Julian Whitaker's Health and Healing* 3, no. 9 (supplement) (September 1993): 2.

6.    Robert McCaleb, "Herbs in Your Medicine Chest," *Energy Times* (May/June 1994): 33.

7.    For example, see E. Roberts, "Pregnenolone—From Selye to Alzheimer and a Model of the Pregnenolone Sulfate Binding Site on the GABA Receptor," *Biochemical Pharmacology* 49 (1995): 1–16; and R. Davison et al., "Effects of delta 5 Pregnenolone in Rheumatoid Arthritis," *Archives of Internal Medicine* 85 (1950): 365–88.

8.    Harvey Diamond and Marilyn Diamond, *Fit for Life* (New York: Warner Books, 1985), 90–91.

9.    Donald J. Brown, *Herbal Prescriptions for Better Health* (Rocklin, Calif.: Prima Publishing, 1995), 267.

10.   Jason Theodosakis, Brenda Adderly, and Barry Fox, *The Arthritis Cure* (New York: St. Martin's Press, 1997).

11.   D. D. Palmer, *Chiropractor's Adjuster* (Portland, Oreg.: Portland Printing House, 1910); and Robert A. Leach, *The Chiropractic Theories* (Baltimore, Md.: Williams and Wilkins, 1986).

12.   The page numbers cited in parentheses in this paragraph refer to Alan R. Gaby, *Preventing and Reversing Osteoporosis* (Rocklin, Calif.: Prima Publishing, 1994).

13.   Gaby, *Preventing and Reversing Osteoporosis*, 253–54.

14.   Santillo, *Food Enzymes*, 13.

15.   Donsbach, *Arthritis*, 20.

16.   Leland B. Taylor, Letter to the Editor, *Health Freedom News* (November/December 1997): 54.

17.   Santillo, *Food Enzymes*, 7.

18.   Ibid.

19.   Julian Whitaker, "Stanford No Longer Uses Microwaves to Warm Breast Milk," *Dr. Julian Whitaker's Health and Healing* 3, no. 9 (September 1993): 3.

20.   Ibid.

21.   Barbara Joseph, *My Healing from Breast Cancer* (New Canaan, Conn.: Keats Publishing, 1996), 230.

22.   John R. Lee, *What Your Doctor May Not Tell You About Menopause* (New York: Warner Books, 1996), 35, 330.

23.   Santillo, *Food Enzymes*, 13.

24.   Julian Whitaker, "Enzymes Safely Reduce Inflammation," *Health and Healing* 8, no. 8 (August 1998): 2.

25. Santillo, *Food Enzymes*, 20.

26. Whitaker, "Enzymes Safely Reduce Inflammation," 2.

27. Donsbach, *Arthritis*, 3.

28. Hanna Kroeger, *God Helps Those Who Help Themselves* (Boulder, Colo.: Hanna Kroeger Publications, 1996), 8.

29. Airola, *There Is a Cure for Arthritis*, 63.

30. Ibid., 153.

31. Theodosakis, Adderly, and Fox, *The Arthritis Cure*, 153.

32. Airola, *There Is a Cure for Arthritis*, 154.

33. Dallas Clouatre, *Anti-Fat Nutrients* (San Francisco, Calif.: Pax Publishing, 1995), 35; and D. A. Lopez, R. M. Williams, and K. Miehlke, *Enzymes: The Fountain of Life* (Charleston, S.C.: The Neville Press, 1994), 95.

34. Santillo, *Food Enzymes*, 16; and John A. McDougall and Mary A. McDougall, *The McDougall Plan* (Piscataway, N.J.: New Century Publishers, 1983).

35. M. T. Morter, Jr., "Osteoporosis!!" *The Chiropractic Professional* (May/June 1987); M. T. Morter, Jr., "Protein," *The Chiropractic Professional* (July/August 1987).

36. Lee, *What Your Doctor May Not Tell You*, 182.

37. Kroeger, *God Helps Those Who Help Themselves*, 8.

38. Santillo, *Food Enzymes*, 13; and Viktoras Kulvinskas, *Survival into the 21st Century* (Fairfield, Iowa: Amongod Press, 1975).

39. Santillo, *Food Enzymes*, 13.

40. Lopez, Williams, and Miehlke, *Enzymes*, 19.

41. Ibid., 20.

42. K. Miehlke, "Enzyme Therapy in Rheumatoid Arthritis," *Natural and Holistic Medicine* 1, no. 108 (1988).

43. Lopez, Williams, and Miehlke, *Enzymes*, quote on 180; and Douglas Hunt, "Relief from Rheumatoid Arthritis," *Journal of Longevity Research* 3, no. 6 (1997): 15.

44. Lopez, Williams, and Miehlke, *Enzymes*, 181–83.

45. Ibid., 43, 184, 185; Charles Anderson, "Potent Fighter Developed Against Rheumatoid Arthritis and Osteoarthritis," *Journal of Longevity* 4, no. 11 (1998): 31; E. Howell, *Enzyme Nutrition* (Garden City Park, N.Y.: Avery Publishing Group, 1985); and Hunt, "Relief from Rheumatoid Arthritis," 15.

46. S. Taussig, "The Mechanism of the Physiological Action of Bromelain," *Medical Hypotheses* 6 (1980): 99–104; and A. Cohen et al., "Bromelain Therapy in Rheumatoid Arthritis," *Pennsylvania Medical Journal* 67 (1964): 27–30.

47. Clouatre, *Anti-Fat Nutrients*, 35.

48. Howard F. Loomis, Jr., *Enzymes: The Key to Health* (Madison, Wis.: Grote, 1999), 78.

49. Loomis, *Enzymes: The Key to Health*, 79.

50. A. Cichoke, *Enzymes and Enzyme Therapy* (New Canaan, Conn.: Keats Publishing, 1994) quoted in Hunt, "Relief from Rheumatoid Arthritis," 15; and Lopez, Williams, and Miehlke, *Enzymes*, 95, 182.

51. Raquel Martin, *The Estrogen Alternative: Natural Hormone Therapy with Botanical Progesterone*, 3rd ed. (Rochester, Vt.: Healing Arts Press, 2000), 197–200. See also Dr. Allen B. Astrow, "Rethinking Cancer," *Lancet* (1994); Linda G. Rector-Page, *Healthy Healing: An Alternative Reference* (Soquel, Calif.: Healthy Healing Publications, 1992), 166, 329; and James F. Balch and Phyllis A. Balch, *Prescription for Nutritional Healing* (Garden City Park, N.Y.: Avery Publishing Group, 1990), 214.

52. Ralph W. Moss, *Cancer Therapy: The Independent Consumer's Guide to Non-Toxic Treatment and Prevention* (New York: Equinox Press, 1992). See also Loren Biser, *The Layman's Course on Killing Cancer* (Charlottesville, Va.: The University of Natural Healing, 1992); and Paavo Airola, *How to Get Well* (Phoenix: Health Plus Publishing, 1985), 43, 55–61.

53. L. G. Darlington et al., "Placebo-Controlled, Blind Study of Dietary Manipulation Therapy in Rheumatoid Arthritis," *Lancet* (1986): 236–38; and William E. Catterall, "Rheumatoid Arthritis Is an Allergy," *Arthritis News Today* (1980).

54. Jeffrey S. Bland, Ph.D., *The Inflammatory Disorders* (syllabus) (Gig Harbor, Wash.: HealthComm, Inc., 1997), 167–202.

55. Lauri M. Aesoph, "Super Healers That Beat Arthritis," *Natural Way*, May/June 1997, 62.

56. G. H. Docena et al., "Identification of Casein as the Major Allergenic and Antigenic Protein of Cow's Milk," *Allergy* 52 (1996): 412–16; and Bland, *The Inflammatory Disorders*, 149.

57. Soltanoff, *Natural Healing*, 222, 223.

58. Ibid., 223.

59. W. J. Peumans et al., "Prevalence, Biological Activity and Genetic

Manipulation of Lectins in Foods," *Trends in Food Science Technology* 7, no. 70 (1996): 132–38.

60. Bruce H. Lithell et al., "A Fasting and Vegetarian Diet Treatment Trial of Chronic Inflammatory Disorders," *Acta Dermato-Venereologica* 63 (1983): 397–403.

61. Stephen T. Sinatra, *Optimum Health* (New York: The Lincoln-Bradley Publishing Group, 1996), 209; and Helen Macfarlane, *Diets to Help Arthritis* (San Francisco: HarperCollins Publishers, 1981), 1, 15, 16.

62. Macfarlane, *Diets to Help Arthritis*, 15–19.

63. Diamond and Diamond, *Fit for Life*, 55.

64. Ibid., 57–58; and David L. Lewis, "Henry Ford and the Wayside Inn," *Early American Life* 5 (1978): 5.

65. Diamond and Diamond, *Fit for Life*, 51–52.

66. Herbert M. Shelton, *The Hygienic System*, 22 (San Antonio, Tex.: Dr. Shelton's Health School, 1934).

67. Diamond and Diamond, *Fit for Life*, 53.

68. Judy Lindberg McFarland, *Aging Without Growing Old* (Palos Verdes, Calif.: Western Front, 1997), 29.

69. Macfarlane, *Diets to Help Arthritis*, 119.

70. Dr. Julian Whitaker, "Throwing Out All of God's Pharmacy," *Dr. Julian Whitaker's Health and Healing* 2, no. 7 (June 1992).

71. Santillo, *Food Enzymes*, 13.

72. Christopher Hartman, "An Interview with Elizabeth Baker," *Health Freedom News*, September/October 1996, 10, 11, 13, 61.

73. Judith A. DeCava, *The Real Truth about Vitamins and Antioxidants* (Columbus, Ga.: Brentwood Academic Press, 1996), 160.

74. Sol Grazi and Marie Costa, *SAMe (S-adenosylmethionine)* (Rocklin, Calif.: Prima Publishing, 1999): 66–68; K. D. Rainsford, "Mechanisms of NSAIDs on Joint Destruction in Osteoarthritis," *Agents and Actions* (Supplements) 44 (1993): 39–43; and M. J. Shield, "Anti-Inflammatory Drugs and Their Effects on Cartilage Synthesis and Renal Function," *European Journal of Rheumatology and Inflammation* 13, no. 1 (1993): 7–16.

75. S. R. Williams, *Nutrition and Diet Therapy* (St. Louis, Mo.: Mirror\Mosby, 1985), 516–18.

76. Bland, *The Inflammatory Disorders*, 7.

77. Ibid., 174. See also L. Mayer et al., "Antigen Trafficking in the Intestine," *Annals of the New York Academy of Sciences* 778 (1996): 28–35.

78. Bland, *The Inflammatory Disorders*, 148. See also R. D. Inmann, "Antigens, the Gastrointestinal Tract, and Arthritis," *Nutr Rheumatic Dis* 17, no. 2 (1991): 309–21.

79. Donna Gates, *The Body Ecology* (Atlanta: B.E.D. Publications, 1996), 160–62.

80. Donna Gates, *The Magic of Kefir* (Atlanta: B.E.D. Publications, 1996), 15.

81. Kroeger, *God Helps Those Who Help Themselves*, 110.

82. M. F. R. Sowers et al., "A Prospective Study of Bone Mineral Content and Fracture in Communities with Differential Fluoride Exposure," *American Journal of Epidemiology* 133 (1991): 649–60. See also S. J. Jacobsen et al., "Regional Variation in the Incidence of Hip Fracture Among White Women Aged 65 Years and Older," *Journal of the American Medical Association* 246 (1990): 500–2; H. Jacqmin-Gadda, "Fluorine Concentration in Drinking Water and Fracture in the Elderly," Letter to the Editor, *Journal of the American Medical Association* 273 (1995): 775–76; and Gaby, *Preventing and Reversing Osteoporosis*, 235.

83. B. L. Riggs et al., "Effect of Fluoride Treatment on Fracture Rate in Postmenopausal Women with Osteoporosis," *New England Journal of Medicine* 322 (1990): 802–9.

84. Lee, *What Your Doctor May* Not *Tell You*, 180, 181; L. R. Hedlund and J. C. Gallagher, "Increased Incidence of Hip Fracture in Osteoporotic Women Treated with Sodium Fluoride," *Journal of Bone and Mineral Research* 4 (1989). See also 223–25; C. Danielson et al., "Hip Fractures and Fluoridation in Utah's Elderly Population," *Journal of the American Medical Association* 268 (1992): 746–47; and Gaby, *Preventing and Reversing Osteoporosis*, 235.

85. James F. Balch and Phyllis A. Balch, *Prescription for Nutritional Healing* (Garden City Park, N.Y.: Avery Publishing Group, 1997), 336.

86. *The Merck Manual*, twelfth ed. (Rahway, N.J.: Merck Sharp & Dohme Research Laboratories, 1972), 1710.

87. Balch and Balch, *Prescription for Nutritional Healing*, 25.

88. Ibid., 15.

89. John R. Lee, "The Selling of Fluoridation in America," *The John R. Lee, M.D. Medical Letter* (February 1999): 2. See also P. J. Mullenix et al., "Neurotoxicity of Sodium Fluoride in Rats," *Neurotoxicology and Teratology* 17 (1995): 169–77; and J. Colquhoun, "Fluoridation in New Zealand: New Evidence," *American Laboratory* 17, no. 5 (1985): 66–72 and 17, no. 6 (1985): 98–102.

90. Thomas J. Moore, *Prescription for Disease* (New York: Simon & Schuster, 1998).

## Chapter 3

1. Jeffrey S. Bland, *The Inflammatory Disorders* (Gig Harbor, Wash.: HealthComm, 1997), 278.

2. Barbara Joseph, *My Healing from Breast Cancer* (New Canaan, Conn.: Keats Publishing, 1996), 17.

3. Ralph W. Moss, *Cancer Therapy: The Independent Consumer's Guide to Non-Toxic Treatment and Prevention* (New York: Equinox Press, 1992); and P. M. Albert, "Physiological Effects of Cabbage with Reference to Its Potential as a Dietary Cancer-Inhibitor and Its Use in Ancient Medicine," *Journal of Ethnopharmacology* 9 (1983): 261–72.

4. Jean Carper, *The Food Pharmacy* (New York: Bantam Books, 1989), 151.

5. Bruce Berkowsky, "Cabbage as Food and Medicine," *Health Freedom News* (June 1993): 34.

6. Ibid, 35.

7. Natalie Angier, "Chemicals in Plants May Help Prevent Cancer," *The Atlanta Journal and Constitution*, 14 April 1993.

8. M. B. Grisham, "Oxidants and Free Radicals in Inflammatory Bowel Disease," *Lancet* 344, no. 8926 (September 1994): 859–61. See also R. S. Britton and B. R. Bacon, "Role of Free Radicals in Liver Diseases and Hepatic Fibrosis," *Hepatogastroenterology* 4, no. 4 (1994): 343–48; P. A. Cerutti, "Oxy-Radicals and Cancer," *Lancet* 455, no. 8926 (1994): 862–63; and I. Davies and A. P. Fotheringham, "Lipofuscin—Does It Affect Cellular Performance?" *Experimental Gerontology* 16 (1981): 119–25.

9. Lauri M. Aesoph, "Super Healers that Beat Arthritis," *Natural Way*, May/June 1997, 63.

10. Ibid, 63.

11. Stephen T. Sinatra, *Optimum Health* (New York: The Lincoln-Bradley Publishing Group, 1996), 209.

12. Carper, *The Food Pharmacy*, 167.

13. Aesoph, "Super Healers that Beat Arthritis," 62.

14. M. Gabor, "Pharmacologic Effects of Flavonoids in Blood Vessels," *Angiologica* 9 (1972): 355–74; and L. W. Blau, "Cherry Diet Control for Gout and Arthritis," *Texas Reports in Biology and Medicine* 8 (1950): 309–11.

15. Helen Macfarlane, *Diets to Help Arthritis* (San Francisco: HarperCollins Publishers, 1994), 35.

16. Anthony Sebastian, "Improved Mineral Balance and Skeletal Metabolism in Postmenopausal Women Treated with Potassium Bicarbonate," *New England Journal of Medicine* 330, no. 25 (1994): 1776–81.

17. Hanna Kroeger, *Heal Your Life with Home Remedies and Herbs* (Carlsbad, Calif.: Hay House, 1998), 249.

18. James F. Balch and Phyllis A. Balch, *Prescription for Nutritional Healing* (Garden City Park, N.Y.: Avery Publishing Group, 1997), 27.

19. Paul C. Bragg and Patricia Bragg, *Apple Cider Vinegar Health System* (Santa Barbara, Calif.: Health Science, 1992), 26–29.

20. Jacques de Langre, *Seasalt's Hidden Powers* (Magalia, Calif.: Happiness Press, 1993).

21. Aesoph, "Super Healers that Beat Arthritis," 61.

22. Stuart M. Berger, *How to Be Your Own Nutritionist* (New York: William Morrow, 1987), 186–93.

23. Kurt W. Donsbach, *Arthritis* (Baja, Calif.: The International Institute of Natural Health Sciences, 1981), 12.

24. Ibid., 9.

25. Ibid.

26. Ibid., 12.

27. W. B. Jonas et al., "The Effect of Niacinamide on Osteoarthritis: A Pilot Study," *Inflammation Research* 45 (1996): 330–34.

28. Robert Petal, "Vitamin C and Inflammation," *Medical Biology* 62, no. 88 (1984).

29. G. Krystal et al., "Stimulation of DNA Synthesis by Ascorbate in Cultures of Articular Chondrocytes," *Arthritis and Rheumatism* 25 (1982): 318–25; and D. F. Horrobin et al., "The Regulation of Prostaglandin $E_1$ Formation: A Candidate for One of the Fundamental Mechanisms Involved in the Actions of Vitamin C," *Medical Hypotheses* 5, no. 8 (1979): 849–58.

30. Karen Sullivan and C. Norman Shealy, *The Complete Family Guide to Alternative Medicine* (Springfield, Mo.: The Shealy Institute, 1997).

31. T. E. McAlindon et al., "Do Antioxidant Micronutrients Protect Against the Development and Progression of Knee Arthritis?" *Arthritis and Rheumatism* 39, no. 4 (1996): 648–56.

32. Jane Heimlich, *What Your Doctor Won't Tell You* (New York: HarperCollins Publishers, 1990), 136–228.

33. Nancy Appleton, *Healthy Bones: What You Should Know About Osteoporosis* (Garden City Park, N.Y.: Avery Publishing Group, 1991), 58, 59.

34. Robert Garrison, Jr., *The Nutrition Desk Reference* (New Canaan, Conn.: Keats Publishing, 1997), 242.

35. Appleton, *Healthy Bones*, 58–59.

36. Mona A. Calvo and Youngmee K. Park, "Changing Phosphorus Content of the U.S. Diet: Potential for Adverse Effects on Bone," *Journal of Nutrition* 126 (1996): 1168S–1180S.

37. Appleton, *Healthy Bones*, 58–59.

38. Ibid., 26.

39. Ibid.

40. Elaine N. Marieb, *Human Anatomy and Physiology* (Benjamin/ Cummings Publishing, 1995), table 25.2. See also Gerard J. Tortora and Nicholas P. Anagnostakos, "Minerals Vital to the Body," in *Principles of Anatomy and Physiology*, 5th edition (New York: Harper and Row, 1987), 651.

41. Balch and Balch, *Prescription for Nutritional Healing*, 27.

42. Ibid., 6.

43. Appleton, *Healthy Bones*, 56.

44. Nancy Appleton, *Lick the Sugar Habit* (Garden City Park, N.Y.: Avery Publishing Group, 1996), 26.

45. Ibid, 25–27.

46. Joseph Z. Schneider, "The Calcium to Phosphorus Ratio as Related to Mineral Metabolism," *International Journal of Orthodontists* 16, no. 3 (1930): 277–85.

47. Melvin E. Page and H. Leon Abram, Jr., *Your Body Is Your Best Doctor* (New Canaan, Conn.: Keats Publishing, 1972).

48. Appleton, *Healthy Bones*, 36–37.

49. Alan R. Gaby, *Preventing and Reversing Osteoporosis* (Rocklin, Calif.: Prima Publishing, 1994), 15. See also B. O'Dell and E. Morris, "Relationship of Excess Calcium and Phosphorus to Magnesium Requirement and Toxicity in Guinea Pigs," *Journal of Nutrition* 82 (1963): 175–81; and Garrison, *The Nutrition Desk Reference*, 243.

50. L. Cohen and R. Kitzes, "Infrared Spectroscopy and Magnesium Content of Bone Mineral in Osteoporotic Women," *Israel Journal of Medical Sciences* 27 (1981): 1132–25; and Gaby, *Preventing and Reversing Osteoporosis*, 107.

51. Suzanne M. Snedeker et al., "Effect of Dietary Calcium and Phosphorus Levels on the Utilization of Iron, Copper, and Zinc by Adult Males," *Journal of Nutrition* 112 (1982): 136–43; and Balch and Balch, *Prescription for Nutritional Healing*, 7.

52. Balch and Balch, *Prescription for Nutritional Healing*, 7.

53. Appleton, *Healthy Bones*, 61, 78, 79.

54. Loren Biser, "Is It Possible to Feel Young Again?" *After Everything FAILS Health Report* 4 (October 1999): 2.

55. Gaby, *Preventing and Reversing Osteoporosis*, 105.

56. Balch and Balch, *Prescription for Nutritional Healing*, 8.

57. Appleton, *Lick the Sugar Habit*, 85.

58. G. E. Abraham and H. Grewal, "A Total Dietary Program Emphasizing Magnesium Instead of Calcium: Effect on the Mineral Density of Calcaneus Bone in Postmenopausal Women on Hormonal Therapy," *Journal of Reproductive Medicine* (1990): 503–7, cited in Gaby, *Preventing and Reversing Osteoporosis*, 108.

59. Gaby, *Preventing and Reversing Osteoporosis*, 108, 109.

60. Appleton, *Lick the Sugar Habit*, 27.

61. Ibid., 25. See also Page and Abram, *Your Body Is Your Best Doctor.*

62. Michael F. Holick, "Vitamin D and Bone Health," *Journal of Nutrition* 126 (1996): 1159S–1164S.

63. Bess Dawson-Hughes, "Calcium and Vitamin D Nutritional Needs of Elderly Women," *Journal of Nutrition* 126 (1996): 1165S–1167S.

64. Holick, "Vitamin D and Bone Health," 1159S–1164S.

65. Donsbach, *Arthritis*, 5.

66. Craig Weatherby and Leonid Gordin, *The Arthritis Bible* (Rochester, Vt.: Healing Arts Press, 1999), 122.

67. MacFarlane, *Diets to Help Arthritis*, 34.

68. Mark Movad, "Vitamin E—Useful or Useless?" *Cancer Communication Newsletter* 14, no. 4 (October 1998); Judith A. DeCava, *The Real Truth About Vitamins and Antioxidants* (Columbus, Ga.: Brentwood Academic Press, 1996); J. D. Ratcliff, "For Heart Disease: Vitamin E," *Coronet* 24, no. 6 (October 1948): 27–32; "Natural Vitamin E for Heart Diseases," *Popular Science Digest*, March 1953, 4–6; and Wilfrid E. Shute, "Vitamin E in Preventive Medicine," in *New Dynamics of Preventive Medicine*, ed. Leon R. Pomeroy (New York: Intercontinental Medical Book, 1974), 36–37.

69. DeCava, *The Real Truth About Vitamins*, 89–90.

70. Whitaker, *Dr. Julian Whitaker's Health and Healing*, 2.

71. DeCava, *The Real Truth About Vitamins*.

72. Ezra Levin, "Vitamin E vs. Wheat Germ Oil," *American Journal of Digestive Diseases* 12, no. 1 (1945): 20–21; and DeCava, *The Real Truth About Vitamins*, 121–22.

73. P. E. Phillips, "Viral Arthritis," *Current Opinion in Rheumatology* 4 (1997): 337–44.

74. Whitaker, *Dr. Julian Whitaker's Health and Healing*.

75. Sinatra, *Optimum Health*, 209.

76. Aesoph, "Super Healers that Beat Arthritis," 62.

77. Hanna Kroeger, *God Helps Those Who Help Themselves* (Boulder, Colo.: Hanna Kroeger Publications, 1996), 154.

78. Aesoph, "Super Healers that Beat Arthritis," 63.

79. Gaby, *Preventing and Reversing Osteoporosis*.

80. Ibid., 11.

81. Sol Grazi, *SAMe (S-adenosylmethionine)* (Rocklin, Calif.: Prima Publishing, 1999), 17.

82. Paavo O. Airola, *There Is a Cure for Arthritis* (West Nyack, N.Y.: Parker Publishing Company, 1968), 73.

83. Macfarlane, *Diets to Help Arthritis*, 8.

84. Dallas Clouatre, *Anti-Fat Nutrients* (San Francisco: Pax Publishing, 1995), 150.

85. Elaine Newkirk, "ADHD or Allergy?" *Health Keepers Magazine* 11, no. 11 (Summer 1999).

86. Appleton, *Lick the Sugar Habit*, 99.

87. Woodrow C. Monte, "Aspartame: Methanol and the Public Health," *Journal of Applied Nutrition* 36, no. 1 (November 1984): 41–52, cited in Jane Heimlich, "Why Aspartame Causes Side Effects," *Dr. Julian Whitaker's Health and Healing* 3, no. 1 (January 1993): 6.

88. G. R. Austin, "Nutrasweet: Friend or Foe?" *Back Issues and Nutrition* no. 3 (1993): 2.

89. Dennis W. Remington, *The Bitter Truth About Artificial Sweeteners* (Provo, Utah: Vitality House International, 1987), cited in Jane Heimlich, "Why Aspartame Causes Side Effects," *Dr. Julian Whitaker's Health and Healing* 3, no. 1 (January 1993): 6.

90. Russell L. Blaylock, *Excitotoxins: The Taste That Kills* (Sante Fe, N.M.: Health Press, 1996).

91. Raymond Peat, "Estrogen and Brain Aging in Men and Women," *Ray Peat's Newsletter*, issue 131 (June 1999).

92. A. D. Kinghorn, *Food Ingredient Safety Review, Stevia Rebaudiana Leaves* (Boulder, Colo.: Herb Research Foundation, 1992); and R. Curi et al., "Effect of Stevia Rebaudiana on Glucose Tolerance in Normal Adult Humans," *Brazilian Journal of Medical Research* 19, no. 6 (1986): 771–74.

93. Daniel P. Mowrey, *Scientific Validation of Herbal Medicine* (New Canaan, Conn.: Keats Publishing, 1990).

94. D. D. Soejarto et al., "Potential Sweetening Agents of Plant Origin," *Economic Botany* 37, no. 1 (1983): 71–79.

95. *Magic and Medicine of Plants* (Pleasantville, N.Y.: Reader's Digest, 1986), 390.

96. MacFarlane, *Diets to Help Arthritis*, 28.

97. Balch and Balch, *Prescription for Nutritional Healing* (1990 ed.), 47.

98. MacFarlane, *Diets to Help Arthritis*, 28.

99. Balch and Balch, *Prescription for Nutritional Healing* (1997 ed.), 25, 77.

100. John Finnegan and Kathy Cituk, *Amazake* (Berkeley, Calif.: Celestial Arts, 1990), 27.

101. Joel Robbins, "Nutrition and Its Relation to Health" (Tulsa, Okla.: Health Dynamics, 1999, cassette).

102. Ibid.

103. Bernard Jensen, *Arthritis, Rheumatism and Osteoporosis: An Effective Program for Correction Through Nutrition* (Escondido, Calif.: Bernard Jensen International, 1986).

104. Carper, *The Food Pharmacy*, 298.

105. Jason Theodosakis, Brenda Adderly, and Barry Fox, *The Arthritis Cure* (New York: St. Martin's Press, 1997), 121.

106. Carper, *The Food Pharmacy*, 186–87, quote on 186.

107. Ibid., 256.

108. Sherry Roger, *Dr. Sherry Roger's Total Health in Today's World* 2, no. 2 (February 1998): 4; and N. F. Childress et al., "An Apparent Relation of Nightshades (Solenacene) to Arthritis," *Journal of Neurological Orthopaedic Medicine and Surgery* 14 (1993): 227–31.

109. Paavo O. Airola, *How to Get Well* (Phoenix: Health Plus Publishers, 1974), 231.

110. Theodosakis, Adderly, and Fox, *The Arthritis Cure*, 107.

111. The Burton Goldberg Group, *Alternative Medicine* (Puyallup, Wash.: Future Medicine Publishing, 1993), 225.

112. James Jamieson and L. E. Dorman, *Growth Hormone: Reversing Human Aging Naturally* (Longevity News Network, 1997).

113. Bland, *The Inflammatory Disorders*, 222.

114. Malkmus, *God's Way to Ultimate Health*, 149.

115. Aesoph, "Super Healers that Beat Arthritis," 63.

116. Macfarlane, *Diets to Help Arthritis*, 31.

117. Aesoph, "Super Healers that Beat Arthritis," 60.

118. D. A. Lewis et al., *International Journal of Crude Drug Research* 23, no. 1 (1985): 27.

119. Jean Carper, *Food—Your Miracle Medicine* (New York: Harper Collins, 1993), 485.

120. Macfarlane, *Diets to Help Arthritis*, 16.

121. N. W. Walker, *Fresh Vegetable and Fruit Juices* (Prescott, Ariz.: Norwalk Press, 1978), 30.

122. Burton Goldberg Group, *Alternative Medicine* (Puyallup, Wash.: Future Medicine Publishing, 1993), 316–18.

123. Bland, *The Inflammatory Disorders*, 27.

124. Malkmus, *God's Way to Ultimate Health*, 148.

125. Aesoph, "Super Healers that Beat Arthritis," 61.

126. Malkmus, *God's Way to Ultimate Health*, 156–59.

127. Raquel Martin and Judi Gerstung, *The Estrogen Alternative: Natural Hormone Therapy with Botanical Progesterone*, 3rd ed. (Rochester, Vt.: Healing Arts Press, 2000), 126–50.

128. Macfarlane, *Diets to Help Arthritis*, 11.

129. Linda G. Rector-Page, *Healthy Healing: An Alternative Reference* (Garden City Park, N.Y.: Healthy Healing Publications, 1992), 166.

130. A. Glenn Braswell, "Letter from the Publisher," *Journal of Longevity*, 4, no. 6 (1998).

131. A. Lietti et al., "Studies on *Vaccinium Myrtillus* Anthocyanosides: Vasoprotective and Anti-Inflammatory Activity," *Arzneim-Forsch Drug Research*, 26, no. 5 (1976): 829–32. See also E. Mian et al., "Anthocyanosides and the Walls of Microvessels: Further Aspects of the Mechanism of Action of their Protective Effect in Syndromes Due to Abnormal Capillary Fragility," *Minerva Medica* 68 (1977): 3565–81; and C. N. Rao et al., "Influence of Bioflavonoids on the Collagen

Metabolism in Rats with Adjuvant Induced Arthritis," *Italian Journal of Biochemistry* 30 (1981): 54–62.

132. Billie J. Sahley, "Boswella: Herb for Arthritis Pain," *The Good Earth News* 14, no. 6 (June/July 1997): 2.

133. G. B. Singh et al., "Pharmacology of an Extract of Salai Guggul Ex-*Boswella Serrata:* A New Non-Steroidal Anti-Inflammatory Agent," *Agents and Actions* 18, no. 3/4 (1986): 407–11. See also G. B. Singh et al., "Boswellic Acids," *Drugs of the Future* 19, no. 4 (1993): 307–9; and V. N. Gupta et al., "Pharmacology of the Gum Resin of *B. Serrata*," *Indian Drugs* 24, no. 5 (1987): 221–23.

134. *Arthritis News* 1 (Summer 1989).

135. "Cat's Claw—A Wonder Herb from the Peruvian Rain Forest," *Newlife*, February 1995.

136. Phillip N. Steinberg, "Uncaria Tomentosa (Cat's Claw): Wonder Herb from the Amazon," *Herb Quarterly* (Winter 1995). See also Phillip N. Steinberg, "Cat's Claw Update (*Uncaria Tomentosa*): That Wondrous Herb from the Peruvian Rain Forest," *Townsend Letter for Doctors* (August/September 1995); M. De Vos, "Articular Diseases and the Gut: Evidence for a Strong Relationship Between Spondylarthropy and Inflammation of the Gut in Man," *Acta Clinica Belgica* 45, no. 1 (1990): 20–24; and M. P. Hazenberg, "Intestinal Flora and Arthritis: Why the Joint?" *Scandinavian Journal of Rheumatology* 24 (supplement 101) (1995): 207–11.

137. Patricia Andersen-Parrado, "Scratching the Surface of Cat's Claw's Health-Promoting Capabilities," *Better Nutrition*, September 1997, 24.

138. Ibid.

139. Phillip N. Steinberg, "Uncaria Tomentosa (Cat's Claw) a Wondrous Herb from the Peruvian Rain Forest," *Townsend Letter for Doctors*, May 1994; and Phillip N. Steinberg, "Uncaria Tomentosa (Cat's Claw): Wonder Herb from the Amazon."

140. Phillip N. Steinberg, "Cat's Claw Update (*Uncaria Tomentosa*): That Wondrous Herb from the Peruvian Rain Forest." See also Don Sanchez, "Cat's Claw," *New Editions Health World*, December 1995, 40–45; and Mark Blumenthal, "Una de Gato (Cat's Claw): Rain Forest Herb Gets Scientific and Industry Attention," *Whole Foods Magazine*, October 1995.

141. Donald J. Brown, *Herbal Prescriptions for Better Health* (Rocklin, Calif.: Prima Publishing 1995), 267.

142. R. Kampf, *Schweizerische Apotheker-Zeitung* 114 (1976): 337–42.

143. M. Pinget, "The Effects of Harpagophytum Capsules (Arkocaps) in Degenerative Rheumatology," 12, no. 4 (1985): 65–67; and C. Dahout, *Journal de Pharmacie de Belgique* 35, no. 2 (1980): 143–49.

144. Hildegard Pickles, *Devil's Claw or Harpagophytum Procumbens: Its Remarkable Medicinal Properties*, (Reforma AG, Postfach, 630 Zug Switzerland), 6, 7.

145. Victoria Dolby, "Devil's Claw: 'Angelic' Relief for Arthritis," *Better Nutrition* 59, no. 6 (June 1997): 3.

146. S. D. Deodhar, "Preliminary Study on Antirheumatic Activity on Curcumin (Diferuloyl Methane)," *Indian Journal of Medical Research* 71 (1980): 632–34.

147. For information on ginger's joint-mending capabilities, see Aesoph, "Super Healers that Beat Arthritis," 62; and K. C. Srivastava and T. Mustafa, "Ginger in Rheumatism and Musculo Skeletal Disorders," *Medical Hypotheses* 39 (1992): 342–48. For information on ginger's ability to inhibit prostaglandins, see Aesoph, "Super Healers that Beat Arthritis," 62. For information on ginger as an anti-inflammatory, see Debbie Moskowitz, "Oh My Aching . . . Joints," *Natural* V, no. 1 (Winter 1997): 1.

148. K. C. Srivastava et al., "Ginger (Zingiber Officinale) and Rheumatic Disorders," *Medical Hypotheses* 29, no. 1 (1989): 25–28; and Srivastava and Mustala, "Ginger in Rheumatism," 342–48.

149. Weatherby and Gordin, *The Arthritis Bible*, 129.

150. Andrew Weil, *8 Weeks to Optimum Health* (New York: Alfred A. Knopf, 1997), 117.

151. Sinatra, *Optimum Health*, 209.

152. N. Peerzoda et al., "Vitamin C and Elemental Composition of Some Bushfruits," *Journal of Plant Nutrition* 13, no. 7 (1990): 787.

153. Riga Elkins, *Noni (Morinda Citrifolia)* (Pleasant Grove, Utah: Woodland Publishing, 1997), 6.

154. Ibid., 23.

155. Ibid., 21.

156. Ibid., 22.

157. Ibid., 11.

158. N. G. Bisset, "*Salicis Cortex*: Willow Bark," in *Herbal Drugs and Phytopharmaceuticals: A Handbook for Practice on a Scientific Basis* (Stuttgart: Medpharm Scientific Publishers, 1994), 437–39, cited in Jeffrey S. Bland, "Phytonutrition, Phytotherapy, and Phytopharmacology," *Alternative Therapies in Health and Medicine* 2, no. 6 (1996); and

Julian Whitaker, "Herbal Pain Relievers," *Dr. Julian Whitaker's Health and Healing* 8, no. 5 (May 1998): 7.

159. For information on the side effects of nausea, see Joe Graedon, *The People's Pharmacy* (New York: Avon Books, 1977).

160. Ibid., 5, 127.

161. Gaby, *Preventing and Reversing Osteoporosis*, 194. See also W. D. Kaehney, "Newer Understanding of Aluminum Metabolism," *Immunology* 6, no. 6 (1985): 131–40.

162. Nicola Giacona and the editors of *Consumer Guide, Prescription Drugs* (Skokie, Ill.: Publications International, 1987), 688.

163. Andrew Weil, *Health and Healing* (Boston: Houghton Mifflin, 1985), 68.

164. *The Magic and Medicine of Plants* (New York: Readers Digest, 1993), 333.

165. M. Blumenthal et al., *The Complete German Commission E Monographs: Therapeutic Guides to Herbal Medicine. Willow Bark* (Boston: American Botanical Council/Integrative Medicine Communications, 1998), 230, cited in Weatherby and Gordin, *The Arthritis Bible*, 137.

166. James F. Balch and Phyllis A. Balch, *Prescription for Nutritional Healing* (Garden City Park, N.Y.: Avery Publishing Group, 1997), 79.

167. Aesoph, "Super Healers that Beat Arthritis," 62.

168. The Burton Goldberg Group, *Alternative Medicine* (Puyallup, Wash.: Future Medicine Publishing, 1993), 533, 534; and R. Bingham, "Yucca Extract," *The Journal of the Academy of Rheumatoid Diseases* 2, no. 1 (1990): 20.

169. Balch and Balch, *Prescription for Nutritional Healing*, 79.

170. Dallas Clouatre, *Anti-Fat Nutrients* (San Francisco: Pax Publishing, 1995), 35; and J. M. Miller et al., *Experimental Medicine and Surgery* 22 (1964): 293–99.

171. R. B. Arora et al., "Anti-Inflammatory Studies on Curcuma Longa (Turmeric)," *Indian Journal of Medicine* 59 (1971): 1289–95; and Julian Whitaker, "An Arthritis Program That's Better than Conventional Treatment," *Dr. Julian Whitaker's Health and Healing* 7, no. 8 (August 1997): 5.

172. H. C. Korting et al., "Anti-inflammatory Activity of Hamamelis Distillate Applied Topically to the Skin," *European Journal of Clinical Pharmacology* 44 (1993): 315–18.

173. L. J. Leventhal et al., "Treatment of Rheumatoid Arthritis with Black Current Seed Oil," *British Journal of Rheumatology* 33 (1994): 847–52.

174. Whitaker, "An Arthritis Program That's Better than Conventional Treatment," 5; and Julian Whitaker, "At-a-Glance Guide to Using Herbs," *Dr. Julian Whitaker's Health and Healing* 9, no.1 (supplement): 6.

175. Aesoph, "Super Healers That Beat Arthritis," 34.

176. Ann M. Fletcher, *Eat Fish, Live Better,* (New York: Harper and Row, 1989).

177. Aesoph, "Super Healers That Beat Arthritis," 60.

178. Ibid, 62.

179. M. Patrick et al., "Feverfew in Rheumatoid Arthritis: A Double-Blind Placebo Controlled Study," *Annals of the Rheumatic Diseases* 48, no. 7 (1989): 547–49.

180. Aesoph, "Super Healers That Beat Arthritis," 60.

181. T. Bodi, *Clinical Medicine* 73 (1966): 61–65.

182. Aesoph, "Super Healers That Beat Arthritis," 62, 63.

183. Jensen, *Arthritis, Rheumatism and Osteoporosis,* 59.

184. Patricia Anderson-Parrado, "Homeopathic Remedies to Ease Acute and Chronic Arthritis Pain," *Better Nutrition* 159, no. 2 (February 1997): 26.

185. Andrew Weil, *Health and Healing* (Boston: Houghton Mifflin, 1985), 14, 17, 18; and Frank L. King, "Homeopathy—a True Sister of Chiropractic," *The Chiropractic Journal* 4, no. 6 (March 1990): 25.

186. Andrew Weil, *Health and Healing;* Emanuel Swedenborg, *Arcana Coelestia* (New York: Swedenborg Foundation, 1961).

187. Eustace Mullins, *Murder by Injection: The Story of the Medical Conspiracy Against America* (Staunton, Va.: National Council for Medical Research, 1988), 1.

188. Paavo O. Airola, *Handbook of Natural Healing* (Sherwood, Oreg.: Health Plus Publishers, 1993), 24.

## Chapter Four

1. John Finnegan, "Our Need for Essential Fatty Acids," *Health Freedom News,* January-February 1997, 34.

2. John Finnegan, *The Facts About Fats* (Berkeley: Celestial Arts, 1993).

3. P. S. Tappia et al., "Influence of Unsaturated Fatty Acids on the Production of Tumor Necrosis Factor and Interleukin-6 by Rat Peritoneal Macrophages," *Molecular and Cellular Biochemistry* 143, no. 2 (1995): 89–98; and C. W. Welsch, "Review of the Effects of Dietary Fat on Experimental Mammary Gland Tumorigenesis: Role of Lipid Peroxidation," *Free Radical Biology and Medicine* 18, no. 4 (1995): 757–73.

4.  Raymond H. Peat, *From PMS to Menopause: Female Hormones in Context* (Eugene, Oreg.: International University, 1997): 155–56. See also E. A. Mascioli et al.,"Unsaturated Fats Directly Kill White Blood Cells," *Lipids* 22, no. 6 (1987): 421; C. J. Meade and J. Martin, "Fatty Acids and Immunity," *Advances in Lipid Research* (1978): 127; and Raymond H. Peat, "Unsaturated Vegetable Oils: Toxins," *Ray Peat's Newsletter* (1997): 3–4.

5.  Udo Erasmus, *Fats that Heal, Fats that Kill* (Vancouver, B.C., Canada: Alive Books, 1997), 103.

6.  Simone Gabbay, "Dietary Fats: The Good and the Bad," *Venture Inward*, May/June 1997, 15.

7.  Erasmus, *Fats that Heal, Fats that Kill*, 98.

8.  Dallas Clouatre, *Anti-Fat Nutrients* (San Francisco: Pax Publishing, 1995), 61. See also P. A. Southorn and G. Powis, "Free Radicals in Medicine I: Chemical Nature and Biologic Reactions," *Mayo Clinic Proceedings* 63 (1988): 381–89; and P. A. Southorn and G. Powis, "Free Radicals in Medicine II: Involvement in Human Disease," *Mayo Clinic Proceedings* 63 (1988): 390–408.

9.  Peat, *From PMS to Menopause*, 153.

10. C. V. Felton et al., "Dietary Polyunsaturated Fatty Acids and Composition of Human Aortic Plaques," *Lancet* 344, no. 8931 (1994): 1195–96; and H. G. P. Swarts et al., "Binding of Unsaturated Fatty Acids to Na+,K+-ATPase Leading to Inhibition and Inactivation," *Biochimica et Biophysica Acta* 1024 (1990): 32–40.

11. Mascioli et al., "Unsaturated Fats Directly Kill White Blood Cells," 421.

12. B. Barnes and L. Galton, *Hypothyroidism: The Unsuspected Illness*, (New York: Harper and Row, 1976), 308. See also Peat, *From PMS to Menopause*, 178; and Sanchez Olea et al., "Inhibition by Polyunsaturated Fatty Acids of Cell Volume Regulation and Osmolyte Fluxes in Astrocytes," *American Journal of Physiology: Cell Physiology* 38, no. 1 (1995): C96–C102.

13. C. F. Aylsworth et al., "Effect of Fatty Acids on Junctional Communication: Possible Role in Tumor Promotion by Dietary Fat," *Lipids* 22, no. 6 (1987): 445–54. See also I. A. Kudryavtsev et al., "Character of the Modifying Action of Polyunsaturated Fatty Acids on Growth of Transplantable Tumors of Various Types," *Bulletin of Experimental Biology and Medicine* 105, no. 4 (1986): 567–70; and Tappia et al., "Influence of Unsaturated Fatty Acids," 89–98.

14. J. K. G. Kramer et al., *Lipids* 17 (1983): 372.

15. Meade and Martin, "Fatty Acids and Immunity," 127–65.

16. Erasmus, *Fats that Heal, Fats that Kill*, 355.

17. Ibid.

18. Dallas Clouatre, Ph.D., tells us that sugar is a "deadly enemy" to our health. When refined, sugar severely "disturbs the metabolism of minerals, insulin and lipids." Clouatre, *Anti-Fat Nutrients*, 137.

19. Peat, *From PMS to Menopause*. See also Meade and Martin, "Fatty Acids in Immunity," 127.

20. Clouatre, *Anti-Fat Nutrients*, 62. See also Sandra Goodman, *Vitamin C: The Master Nutrient* (New Canaan, Conn.: Keats Publishing, 1991).

21. Clouatre, *Anti-Fat Nutrients*, 18.

22. Elson Haas, *Staying Healthy* (Berkeley, Calif.: Celestial Arts, 1992); and California Avocado Commission, "Avocados," *Energy Times*, September 1998, 18.

23. Julian M. Whitaker, *99 Secrets for a Longer Healthier Life* (Potomac, Md.: Phillips Publishing, 1992), 17.

24. Clouatre, *Anti-Fat Nutrients*, 137.

25. Robert S. Goodhart and Maurice E. Shils, *Modern Nutrition in Health and Disease*, 8th ed. (Baltimore, Md.: Williams and Wilkins, 1994).

26. Eustace Mullins, *Murder by Injection: The Story of the Medical Conspiracy Against America* (Staunton, Va.: The National Council for Medical Research, 1988), 214.

27. William G. Crook, *The Yeast Connection* (New York: Random House, 1986). See also Mascioli et al.,"Unsaturated Fats Directly Kill White Blood Cells," 421; and Meade and Martin, "Fatty Acids and Immunity," 127.

28. Peat, *From PMS to Menopause*; and Welsch, "Review of the Effects of Dietary Fat," 757–73. See also K. L. Erickson et al., "Dietary Lipid Modulation of Immune Responsiveness," *Lipids* 18 (1983): 468–74; D. Harman et al., "Free Radical Theory of Aging: Effect of Dietary Fat on Central Nervous System Function," *Journal of the American Geriatrics Society* 24, no. 1 (1976): 292–98; and M. L. Pearce and S. Dayton, "Incidence of Cancer in Men on a Diet High in Polyunsaturated Fat," *Lancet* 1 (1971): 464–67.

29. H. Selye, "Sensitization by Corn Oil for the Production of Cardiac Necrosis," *American Journal of Cardiology* 23 (1969): 719–22. See also Erickson et al., "Dietary Lipid Modulation of Immune Responsiveness," 468–74; and Jane Heimlich, "What the Food Industry Won't Tell You About Margarine and Other Man-Made Fats," *Dr. Julian Whitaker's Health and Healing* 1, no. 3 (October 1991): 6, 7.

30. D. A. Lopez, R. M. Williams, and K. Miehlke, *Enzymes: The Fountain of Life* (Salem, Mass.: Neville Press, 1994), 218.

31. Julian Whitaker, *Dr. Julian Whitaker's Health and Healing* 7, no. 10 (October 1997): 4; and M. G. Enig, "Trans Fatty Acids—An Update," *Nutrition Quarterly* 17, no. 4 (1993): 79–95.

32. Goodman, *Vitamin C: The Master Nutrient*, and Clouatre, *Anti-Fat Nutrients*, 62.

33. Erasmus, *Fats that Heal, Fats that Kill*, 95–97.

34. Ibid., 399

35. Ibid., 96.

36. Ibid., 97.

37. Gabbay, "Dietary Fats: The Good and the Bad," 15.

38. Clouatre, *Anti-Fat Nutrients*, 17.

39. Whitaker, *Dr. Julian Whitaker's Health and Healing* 7, no. 10, 4.

40. Selye, "Sensitization by Corn Oil," 719–22.

41. Peat, *From PMS to Menopause*, 153–57, 178, 180.

42. Matthew Gillman, "Beyond Cholesterol: A New Heart Attack Predictor," *Health*, July/August 1997.

43. Erasmus, *Fats that Heal, Fats that Kill*, 106.

44. Whitaker, *Dr. Julian Whitaker's Health and Healing*, 4; and R. P. Mensink et al., "Effect of Dietary Trans Fatty Acids on High-Density and Low-Density Lipoprotein Cholesterol Levels in Healthy Subjects," *New England Journal of Medicine* 323 (1990): 439–45.

45. Erasmus, *Fats That Heal, Fats That Kill*, 125.

46. Peat, "Unsaturated Vegetable Oils: Toxic," 3.

47. Peat, *From PMS to Menopause*, 154–55. See also Wolfe, *J Am Oil Chem Soc*, 230; and Wolfe (Chem 121, University of Oregon, 1986).

48. Peat, *From PMS to Menopause*, 157, 180.

49. William Campbell Douglass, "Coconut Oil Slows Aging and Weight Gain," *Second Opinion* VIII, no. 4 (April 1998): 2.

50. Ibid, 4.

51. Peat, *From PMS to Menopause*, 177. See also F. Berschauer et al., "Nutritional-Physiological Effects of Dietary Fats in Rations for Growing Pigs: Effects of Sunflower Oil and Coconut Oil on Protein and Fat Retention, Fatty Acid Pattern of Back Fat and Blood Parameters in Piglets," *Archiv Fur Tierernahrung* 34, no. 2 (1984): 19–33.

52. Peat, *From PMS to Menopause*, 179–81.

53. Ibid., 153. See also Kramer et al., 372.

54. Peat, *From PMS to Menopause*, 157.

55. Ibid., 161.

56. Anne Dolamone, *The Essential Olive Oil Companion* (New York: Interlink Books, 1994), 32, 52–53, 156.

57. Raymond H. Peat, "Unsaturated Vegetable Oils: Toxic," *Ray Peat's Newsletter*, 3, 4.

58. Erasmus, *Fats That Heal, Fats That Kill*, 256–57.

59. Ibid., 257–58.

60. Barbara Joseph, *My Healing from Breast Cancer* (New Canaan, Conn.: Keats Publishing, 1996), 150.

61. Jason Theodosakis, Brenda Adderly, and Barry Fox, *The Arthritis Cure* (New York: St. Martin's Press, 1997), 120.

62. Susan Smith Jones, *The Main Ingredients of Health and Happiness* (Dawn Publications, 1995).

63. Peat, *From PMS to Menopause*, 157; and M. Jenab and L. U. Thompson, *Carcinogenesis* 17, no. 1343 (1996).

64. Jeffrey S. Bland, *The Inflammatory Disorders* (Gig Harbor, Wash.: HealthComm, 1997), 275.

65. Ibid.

66. R. Chopra, et al., "Relative Bioavailability of Coenzyme Q10 Formulations in Human Subjects," *International Journal for Vitamin and Mineral Research*, 1998 cited in S. Sinatra, "CoQ10 Formulation Can Influence Bioavailability," *Nutrition Science News* 2, no. 2 (1997): 88.

67. Clouatre, *Anti-Fat Nutrients*, 61.

68. Sally W. Fallon and Mary G. Enig, "Why Butter Is Better," *Health Freedom News* 14, no. 6 (November/December 1995): 12–14. See also J. J. Kabara, *The Pharmacological Effects of Lipids* (Champaign, Ill.: The American Oil Chemists Society, 1978), 1–14.

69. Fallon and Enig, "Why Butter Is Better," 14; and Kabara, *The Pharmacological Effects of Lipids*, 1–14.

70. Fallon and Enig, "Why Butter Is Better," 14.

71. Ibid.

72. Cheryl Player, "Ghee: An Ancient Food for a Modern Era," *A Grain of Salt*, Spring 1999, 2. See also K. Feldenkreis, *Ghee—A Guide to the Royal Oil* (Kearney, Nebr.: Morris Publishing, 1996); P. Pritchford,

*Healing with Whole Foods* (Berkeley, Calif.: North Atlantic Books, 1993); and V. Lad, *The Complete Book of Ayurvedic Home Remedies* (New York: Harmony Books, 1998).

73. Heimlich et al., "Effect of Dietary Enrichment with Eicosapentaenoic and Docosahexaenoic Acids in Vitra Neutrophil and Monocyte Leukotriene Generation and Neutrophil Function," *New England Journal of Medicine* 312 (1985): 146.

74. Julian Whitaker, *147 Medically-Proven Miracle Cures* (Potomac, Md.: Phillips Publishing, 1996), 7; and Theodosakis, Adderly, and Fox, *The Arthritis Cure*, 120.

75. Joel M. Kremer et al., "Effects of Manipulation of Dietary Fatty Acids on Clinical Manifestations of Rheumatoid Arthritis," *Lancet* 2, no. 840 (1985): 184–87.

76. W. L. Blok et al., "Modulation of Inflammation and Cytokine Production by Dietary (n-3) Fatty Acids," *Journal of Nutrition*, 126 (1996): 1515–33.

77. Erasmus, *Fats that Heal, Fats that Kill*, 259.

78. AIM, "Is Fish Oil Fishy," *Partners*, September 1998, 12.

79. Jean Carper, *The Food Pharmacy* (New York: Bantam Books, 1989), 53.

80. For information on trout, see Carper, *The Food Pharmacy*, 321. For information on tuna, see Carol H. Munson and Diane K. Gilroy, *The Good Fats* (Emmaus, Pa.: Rodale Press, 1988).

81. Erasmus, *Fats that Heal, Fats that Kill*, 218.

82. Anne M. Fletcher, *Eat Fish, Live Better* (New York: Harper and Row, 1989).

83. A. A. Nanji et al., "Effect of Type of Dietary Fat and Ethanol on Antioxidant Enzyme mRNA Induction in Rat Ethanol Rat Liver," *Journal of Lipid Research* 36, no. 4 (1995): 736–44.

84. Heimlich, *What Your Doctor Won't Tell You*, 148.

85. Ibid., 134.

86. Natural Factor's halibut-liver oil is an excellent source. Available through Seattle Super Supplements, (800) 249-9394.

87. Erasmus, *Fats that Heal, Fats that Kill*, 354.

88. Sherrie Schatz and Sheree Lewis, "Emu Oil: Reexamining a Natural Remedy with Today's Technology," *Emu Today and Tomorrow* (1996): 29–35.

89. Sheree Lewis, "An Active Ingredient: Elusive Anti-Inflammatory Component of Emu Oil Isolated," *Emu Today and Tomorrow* 5, no. 10 (October 1995): 46.

90. Schatz and Lewis, "Emu Oil: Reexamining a Natural Remedy with Today's Technology," 38.

91. Lewis, "An Active Ingredient: Elusive Anti-Inflammatory Component of Emu Oil Isolated," 46.

92. Beth Silva, "Emu Oil Is This Physician's Choice," *Emu Today and Tomorrow* 8, no. 10 (October 1998): 3.

93. Craig Weatherby and Leonid Gordin, *The Arthritis Bible* (Rochester, Vt.: Healing Arts Press, 1999), 250.

94. Sheree Lewis, *Emu Today and Tomorrow* 7, no. 10 (October 1997): 3.

95. Ibid., 1–2.

96. Heimlich, *What Your Doctor Won't Tell You*, 78.

97. Fallon and Enig, "Is the Bad Guy Really Good?" *Health Freedom News* (1996): 24.

98. Finnegan, "Our Need for Essential Fatty Acids," 35. See also Ann Louis Gittleman, *Beyond Pritikin* (New York: Bantam, 1989); Rudolph Ballentine, "Butter vs. Oil," *East/West Journal*, (February 1988); Bruce Alberts et al., *Molecular Biology of the Cell* (New York: Garland, 1989); Robert B. Gennis, *Biomembranes: Molecular Structure and Function* (New York: Springer-Verlag, 1989); and Charles Bates, *Essential Fatty Acids and Immunity in Mental Health* (Washington, D.C.: Life Sciences Press, 1987).

99. Sally W. Fallon and Mary G. Enig, "Our Friend Cholesterol: Is the 'Bad' Guy Really a Good Guy?" *Health Freedom News* (April/May 1996): 24.

100. Lopez, Williams, and Miehlke, *Enzymes: The Fountain of Life*, 217.

101. Hyman Engelberg, *Lancet* 339 (1992): 727–28; cited in Fallon, and Enig, "Our Friend Cholesterol," 24–26.

102. William Regelson and Carol Colman, *The Super-Hormone Promise* (New York: Simon & Schuster, 1996), 103.

103. Fallon and Enig, "Our Friend Cholesterol," 26. and Kabara, *The Pharmacological Effects of Lipids*, 1–14.

104. Charles J. Hunt, *Diet Evolution: Eat Fat and Get Fit* (Beverly Hills, Calif.: Maximum Human Potential Productions, 1999).

105. Fallon and Enig, "Our Friend Cholesterol," 24.

106. Cathy Pinckney and Edward R. Pinckney, *The Patient's Guide to Medical Tests* (New York: Facts on File Publishers, 1986), 83–85; Richard Passwater, *The New Supernutrition* (New York: Simon & Schuster, 1991); and Stephen Langer, *Solved: The Riddle of Illness* (New Canaan, Conn.: Keats Publishing 1995), 99.

107. John R. Lee, "Do Cholesterol-Lowering Drugs Increase Breast Cancer Rate?" *The John R. Lee, M.D. Medical Letter* (March 1999): 4.

108. Bland, *The Inflammatory Disorders*, 216.

109. Fallon and Enig, "Our Friend Cholesterol," 25; and Chris Mudd, *Cholesterol and Your Health* (Oklahoma City, Okla.: American Lite, 1990).

110. *American Botanical Pharmacy News* 2 (1998).

111. Earl L. Mindell, "Eggs Have Gotten a Raw Deal," *Let's Live*, September 1994, 8.

112. Judy Lindberg McFarland, *Aging Without Growing Old* (Palos Verdes, Calif.: Western Front, 1997), 166.

113. Mindell, "Eggs Have Gotten a Raw Deal," 8.

114. Raymond Peat, *Nutrition for Women* (Lake Oswego, N.Y.: Cenotech, 1981), 18, 67, 68, 92.

115. Lloyd Guth et al., "Key Role for Pregnenolone in Combination Therapy that Promotes Recovery After Spinal Cord Injury," *Proceedings of the National Academy of Sciences* 91 (1994): 12308–12.

116. Finnegan, "Our Need for Essential Fatty Acids," 34–35.

117. Patricia Clarke, "Bone/Joint Problems—Can You Expect More Than Relief?" *Journal of Longevity* 5, no. 8 (1999): 18.

## Chapter Five

1. Andrew Weil, *Health and Healing* (Boston: Houghton Mifflin, 1985), 127.

2. John W. Tintera and Delos Smith, "What You Should Know About Your Glands," *Woman's Day*, February 1958. See also H. A. Kurvers et al., "The Spinal Component to Skin Blood Flow Abnormalities in Reflex Sympathetic Dystrophy," *Archives of Neurology* 53, no. 1 (1996): 58–65; and Karen Feeley Collins and Bruce Pfleger, "The Neurophysiological Evaluation of the Subluxation Complex: Documenting the Neurological Component with Somatosensory Potentials," *Chiropractic Research Journal* 3, no. 1 (1994).

3. Tedd Koren, *Arthritis and Chiropractic* (pamphlet) (Philadelphia: Koren Publications, 1989). See also Brian M. Sheres, "Chiropractic Efficacy Progress Report: Treatment of Spinal Neuralgia, Cephalgia, Vertigo and Related Peripheral Conditions," *Chiropractic Research Journal* 2, no. 3 (1993); and J. C. Fidelibus, "An Overview of Neuroimmunomodulation and a Possible Correlation with Musculoskeletal System Function," *Journal of Manipulative and Physiological Therapeutics* 12, no. 4 (1989): 289–92.

4.    G. Waddell, "Chronic Low-Back Pain, Psychologic Distress, and
      Illness Behavior," *Spine* 9, no. 2 (1984): 209–13. See also W. H.
      Quigley, "Physiological Psychology of Chiropractic in Mental
      Disorder," in *Mental Health and Chiropractic: A Multidisciplinary
      Approach* (New Hyde Park, N.Y.: Sessions Publishers, 1973); and H. S.
      Schwartz, "Preliminary Analysis of 350 Mental Patients' Records
      Treated by Chiropractors," *Journal of National Chiropractic Association*
      (November 1949): 12–15.

5.    O. J. Ressel, "Disc Regeneration: Reversability Is Possible in Spinal
      Osteoarthritis," *International Review of Chiropractic* (March/April
      1989): 39–61 cited in Tedd Koren, *Arthritis and Chiropractic* (pam-
      phlet) (Philadelphia: Koren Publications, 1989), 2.

6.    *Primer on the Rheumatic Diseases*, ninth ed. (Atlanta: Arthritis Founda-
      tion, 1988).

7.    Gerard J. Tortora and Nicholas P. Anagnostakos, "Minerals Vital to
      the Body," in *Principles of Anatomy and Physiology*, 5th ed. (New York:
      Harper and Row, 1987), 651.

8.    B. S. Polkinghorn and C. J. Colloca, "Treatment of Symptomatic Lumbar
      Disc Herniation Utilizing Activator Methods Chiropractic Technique,"
      *Journal of Manipulative and Physiological Therapeutics.*

9.    For information on precise adjustments, see M. W. Youngquist, A. W.
      Fuhr, and P. J. Osterbauer, "Interexaminer Reliability of an Isolation
      Test for the Presence of an Upper Cervical Isolation Subluxation,"
      *Journal of Manipulative and Physiological Therapeutics* 12 (1989): 93–97;
      and John D. Grostic, "The Adjusting Instrument as a Research Tool,"
      *Chiropractic Research Journal* 1, no. 2 (1988). For information on the
      communication between the central nervous system and cells, see N. J.
      Phillips, "Vertebral Subluxation and Otitis Media: A Case Study,"
      *Chiropractic* 8, no. 2 (1992): 38–39; Raquel Martin, *Today's Health
      Alternative* (Bozeman, Mont.: America West Publishers, 1992); and
      D. D. Palmer, Palmer College of Chiropractic, *Chiropractor's Adjuster*
      (Portland, Oreg.: Portland Printing House, 1910).

10.   American Chiropractic Association, "Which of These Doctors Are
      Chiropractors?" *Reader's Digest*, (supplement), April 1988; and Louis
      Sportelli, *Introduction to Chiropractic*, 8th ed. (Palmerton, Pa.: n.p.,
      1986), 2.

11.   Jon Mastrobattista, Letter to the Editor, *The Internist* 2, no. IV (1995): 4.

12.   C. Hviid, "A Comparison of the Effects of Chiropractic Treatment on
      Respiratory Function in Patients with Respiratory Distress Symptoms
      and Patients Without," *Bulletin of the European Chiropractic Union* 26
      (1978): 17–34.

13. Stuart M. Berger, *What Your Doctor* Didn't *Learn in Medical School* (New York: William Morrow, 1988), 310, 311.

14. Edward McDonagh, "Can Chiropractic Reverse Osteoporosis?" *The Internist* 2, no. IV (1995): 17–18.

15. James F. Fries, "America's Other Drug Problem," *Los Angeles Times Magazine*, 29 September 1996.

16. Kathryn T. Hoiris et al., "Design and Implementation of a Randomized Controlled Trial of Chiropractic Care Versus Drug Therapy for Sub-Acute Low Back Pain," *Chiropractic Research Journal* 4, no. 2 (1997); and V. Dabbs and W. J. Lauretti, "A Risk Assessment of Cervical Manipulation vs. NSAIDs for the Treatment of Neck Pain," *Journal of Manipulative and Physiological Therapeutics* 18, no. 8 (1995): 530–36.

17. Fidelibus, "An Overview of Neuroimmunomodulation"; F. M. Purse, "Manipulative Therapy of Upper Respiratory Infections in Children," *Journal of the American Osteopathic Association* 65 (1966): 964–71. See also Frank Mechler, "Review of the Anatomy, Histology and Clinical Significance of the Vertebral Artery in Health and Disease," *Chiropractic Research Journal* 1, no. 1 (1988); Kirk Erikson and Edward F. Owens, Jr., "Upper Cervical Post X-Ray Reduction and its Relationship to Symptomatic Improvement and Spinal Stability," *Chiropractic Research Journal* 4, no. 1 (1997); Edward F. Owens et al., "Changes in General Health Status During Upper Cervical Chiropractic Care: PBR Progress Report," *Chiropractic Research Journal* 5, no. 1 (1998); and Sarah K. Webster and Medhat Alattar, "Literature Review: Mechanisms of Physiological Responses to Chiropractic Adjustment," *Chiropractic Research Journal* 6, no. 1 (1998).

18. W. Kunert, "Functional Disorders of Internal Organs Due to Vertebral Lesions," *Ciba Symposium* 13, no. 3 (1965): 88, 96. See also Catherine Parker Anthony and Gary A. Thibodeau, *Anatomy & Physiology*, twelfth ed. (Toronto: Times Mirror/Mosby, 1987), 372; and Webster and Alattar "Literature Review."

19. A. Lanas, et al., "Evidence of Aspirin Use in Both Upper and Lower Gastrointestinal Perforation," *Gastroenterology* 112 (1997): 683–89.

20. J. M. Cox and S. Shreiner, "Chiropractic Manipulation in Low Back Pain and Sciatica; Statistic Data on the Diagnosis, Treatment and Response of 576 Consecutive Cases," *Journal of Manipulative and Physiological Therapeutics* 7, no. 1 (1984): 1–11. See also M. Livingston, "Spinal Manipulation: A One Year Follow-Up Study," *The Canadian Family Physician* 4 (1969): 35–39; J. A. Mathews et al., "Back Pain and Sciatica: Controlled Trials of Manipulation, Traction, Sclerosant and Epidural Injections," *British Journal of Rheumatology* 26 (1987): 416–23;

and U. Herzberg et al., "Spinal Cord NMDA Receptors Modulate Peripheral Immune Responses and Spinal Cord c-fos Expression After Immune Challenge in Rats Subjected to Unilateral Mononeuropathy," *Journal of Neuroscience* 16, no. 2 (1996): 730–43.

21. F. H. Gilles, M. Bina, and A. Sotrel, "Infantile Atlanto-Occipital Instability," *American Journal of Diseases of Children* 133, no. 30 (1979). See also A. Fremion, P. Bhuwan, and J. Kalsbeck, "Apnea as the Sole Manifestation of Cord Compression in Achon Droplasia," *Journal of Pediatrics* 104, no. 3 (1984); and P. N. Sachis et al., "The Vagus Nerve and Sudden Infant Death Syndrome: A Morphometric Study," *Journal of Pediatrics* 98, no. 2 (1981): 278.

22. G. L. Richards et al., "Low Force Chiropractic Care of Two Patients with Sciatic Neuropathy and Lumbar Disc Herniation," *American Journal of Chiropractic Medicine* 3, no. 1 (1990): 25–32. See also J. M. Daly, P. S. Frame, and P. A. Rapoza, "Sacroiliac Subluxation: A Common Treatable Cause of Low Back Pain in Pregnancy," *Family Practice Research Journal* 11, no. 2 (1991): 149–59; and H. E. Fredrick and D. C. Barge, "The Chiropractic Vertebral Subluxation and its Relationship to Vertebrogenic Lumbar Pain, Cruralgia and Sciatic Syndromes," *Chiropractic Research Journal* 3, no. 2 (1996).

23. K. Kokjohn et al., "The Effect of Spinal Manipulation on Pain and Prostaglandin Levels in Women with Primary Dysmenorrhea," *Journal of Manipulative and Physiological Therapeutics* 15, no. 5 (1992): 279–85; Erikson and Owens, "Upper Cervical Post X-Ray Reduction"; and Webster and Alattar, "Literature Review."

24. For information on neck pain, see J. M. McPartland, R. R. Brodeur, and R. C. Hallgren, "Chronic Neck Pain, Standing Balance, and Suboccipital Muscle Atrophy—A Pilot Study," *Journal of Manipulative and Physiological Therapeutics* 20, no. 1 (1997): 24–29; and Dabbs and Lauretti, "A Risk Assessment of Cervical Manipulation," 530–36. For information on knee pain, see Mary Brown and Paul Vaillancourt, "Case Report: Upper Cervical Adjusting for Knee Pain," *Chiropractic Research Journal* 2, no. 4 (1993). For information on shoulder pain, see Rene Cailliet, "Adhesive Capsulitis: The 'Frozen Shoulder,'" *Shoulder Pain* (Philadelphia: F. A. Davis, 1982), 88. For information on other joint pain, see Cox and Shreiner, "Chiropractic Manipulation in Low Back Pain," 1–11.

25. Herbert R. Reaver, "Rebel with a Cause," *Chiropractic Achievers* (March/April 1989): 13–19.

26. Chester A. Wilk et al. v American Medical Association et al., 719 F. 2d 207 (7th Cir. 1983).

27. Ibid.

28. Ibid.

29. Koren, *Arthritis and Chiropractic.*

30. Hviid, "A Comparison of the Effects of Chiropractic Treatment," 17–34; and N. Nilsson and B. Christainson, "Prognostic Factors in Bronchial Asthma in Chiropractic Practice," *Journal of the Australian Chiropractic Association* 18, no. 3 (1988): 85–87.

31. W. M. van Breda, et al., "A Comparative Study of the Health Status of Children Raised Under the Health Care Models of Chiropractic and Allopathic Medicine," *Journal of Chiropractic Research* 5 (1989): 101–3. See also N. H. Nielsen et al., "Chronic Asthma and Chiropractic Spinal Manipulation: A Randomized Clinical Trial," *Clinical and Experimental Allergy* 25, no. 1 (1995): 80–88; Langley, "Epileptic Seizures, Nocturnal Enuresis, ADD (Case Study)," *Chiropractic Pediatrics* 1, no. 1 (1994): 22; Kirby L. Scotty, D.C. "A Case Study: The Effects of Chiropractic on Multiple Sclerosis," *Chiropractic Research Journal* 3, no. 1 (1994); A. A. Pikalov and V. V. Kharin, "Use of Spinal Manipulative Therapy in the Treatment of Duodenal Ulcer: A Pilot Study," *Journal of Manipulative and Physiological Therapeutics* 17, no. 5 (1994): 310–13; and Abraham Towbin, "Latent Spinal Cord and Brain Stem Injury in Newborn Infants," *Developmental Medical Child Neurology* 11 (1969): 54–68.

32. Tony S. Keller, Christopher J. Colloca, and Arlan W. Fuhr, "Validation of the Force and Frequency Characteristics of the Activator Adjusting Instrument: Effectiveness as a Mechanical Impedance Measurement Tool," *Journal of Manipulative and Physiological Therapeutics* 22, no. 2 (1999): 75–86.

33. R. G. Yates et al., "Effects of Chiropractic Treatment on Blood Pressure and Anxiety: A Randomized Controlled Trial," *Journal of Manipulative and Physiological Therapeutics* 11, no. 6 (1988): 484–88. See also M. E. McKnight and K. F. DeBoer, "Preliminary Study of Blood Pressure Changes in Normotensive Subjects Undergoing Chiropractic Care," *Journal of Manipulative and Physiological Therapeutics* 11, no. 4 (1988): 261–66; and Kurvers et al., "The Spinal Component," 58–65.

34. Sachis et al., "The Vagus Nerve," 278. See also Abraham Towbin, "The Pathology of Cerebral Palsy," in *Renaissance Interviews* (Springfield, Ill.: C. C. Thomas, 1960); M. Valdez-Dapena, "A Pathologist's Perspective on Possible Mechanisms in SIDS," *New York Academy of Science* 533 (1988): 31–36; G. B. Giulian, E. F. Gilbert, and R. L. Moss, "Elevated Fetal Hemoglobin Levels in SIDS," *New England*

*Journal of Medicine* 316, no. 18 (1987): 1122–26; and G. F. Vawter and H. Kosakewich, "Aspects of Morphologic Variation Amongst SIDS Victims," in *Sudden Infant Death Syndrome* (New York: Academic Press, 1983), 133–44.

35.  J. M. Giesen, D. B. Center, and R. A. Leach, "An Evaluation of Chiropractic Manipulation as a Treatment of Hyperactivity in Children," *Journal of Manipulative and Physiological Therapeutics* 12, no. 5 (1989): 353–63. See also R. M. Froehle, "Ear Infection: A Retrospective Study Examining Improvement from Chiropractic Care and Analyzing for Influencing Factors," *Journal of Manipulative and Physiological Therapeutics* 19, no. 3 (1996): 169–77; N. J. Phillips, "Vertebral Subluxation and Otitis Media: A Case Study," *Chiropractic* 8, no. 2 (1992): 38–39; and Kirk Eriksen, "Correction of Juvenile Idiopathic Scoliosis After Primary Upper Cervical Chiropractic Care: A Case Study," *Chiropractic Research Journal* 3, no. 3 (1996).

36.  Linda Cook, "The 21st Century: Age of Chiropractic," *Health Freedom News*, Spring 1998, 8.

37.  Ibid.

38.  Tracy A. Barnes, "A Multi-Faceted Chiropractic Approach to Attention Deficit Hyperactivity Disorder: A Case Report," *ICA International Review of Chiropractic* (1995): 41–43; and Tracy A. Barnes, "Attention Deficit Hyperactivity Disorder and The Triad of Health," *Journal of Clinical Chiropractic Pediatrics* 1, no. 2 (1996): 59–65.

39.  K. Gutzeit, "The Vertebral Column as a Factor in Disease," *Deutsche Medizinsche Worchenschrift* 1 (1951): 3–7.

40.  G. Gutman, "Blocked Atlantal Nerve Syndrome in Babies and Infants," *Manuelle Medizin* 25 (1987): 5–10.

41.  David Chapman-Smith, *The Chiropractic Report* 3, no. 2 (1989). See also Gutman, "Blocked Atlantal Nerve Syndrome in Babies and Infants," 5–10; and R. Peters and M. Chance, "A Priceless Legacy; Lost, Strayed or Forfeited," *Australian Chiropractors' Association* 18, no. 3 (1988): 81–84.

42.  Jason Theodosakis, Brenda Adderly, and Barry Fox, *The Arthritis Cure* (New York: St. Martin's Press, 1997), 155.

43.  Ibid., 155, 158.

44.  N. M. Newman et al., "Acetabular Bone Destruction Related to Nonsteroidal Anti-Inflammatory Drugs," *Lancet* 2 (1985): 11–14; and *Scandinavian Journal of Rheumatology* 91 (supplement) (1991): 9–17.

45.  Trien Susan Falmholtz, *Change of Life* (New York: Fawcett Columbine Books, 1986).

46. Barbara Loe Fisher, "Vaccination and Freedom of Conscience," *The American Chiropractor*, (July/August 1993): 8. Seventeen thousand adverse events following vaccinations (including 360 deaths and 2,525 serious injuries) "were reported to the federal government in a twenty-month period ending in July 1992 . . . The FDA estimates only 10 percent of all adverse events . . . are reported by physicians. Therefore, the actual numbers may be 170,000 adverse events following vaccinations, including 3,600 deaths and 25,250 serious injuries." For information on mammograms, see Marcus Laux, "Why I Don't Think You Should Trust Mammograms," *Naturally Well* 3, no. 5 (May 1996), 1–3; W. W. Fletcher, "Why Question Screening Mammography," (1995): 1259–71; Karla Kerlikowski et al., "Efficacy of Screening Mammography: A Meta-Analysis," *Journal of the American Medical Association* 273, no. 2 (1995); Stanley Englebardt, "Straight Talk About Mammograms," *Reader's Digest*, November 1994; Linda G. Rector-Page, *Healthy Healing: An Alternative Reference* (Soquel, Calif.: Healthy Healing Publications, 1992), 166, 329; Maureen Roberts, "Breast Screening: Time for a Rethink?" *British Medical Journal* 299 (1989): 1153–55. For information on medications, see Dee Ito, *Without Estrogen: Natural Remedies for Menopause and Beyond* (New York: Carol Southern Books, 1994), 14.

47. Tintera and Smith, "What You Should Know About Your Glands."

48. Burton Goldberg Group, *Alternative Medicine* (Puyallup, Wash.: Future Medicine Publishing, 1993), 7–8.

49. van Breda et al., "A Comparative Study of the Health Status," 101–3.

50. A. A. Perlik et al., "On the Usefulness of Somato-Sensory Evoked Responses for the Evaluation of Lower Back Pain," *Archives of Neurology* 43 (1986): 907–13.

51. Mechler, "Review of the Anatomy, Histology and Clinical Significance"; and Waddell, "Chronic Low-Back Pain," 209–13.

52. M. T. Morter, Jr., "Osteoporosis!!" *The Chiropractic Professional* (May/June 1987).

53. Emanuel Swedenborg, *Arcana Coelestia* Vol. VIII (New York: Swedenborg Foundation, 1961), 115.

## Chapter Six

1. William Regelson and Carol Colman, *The Super-Hormone Promise* (New York: Simon & Schuster, 1996), 21, 104. See also Alan R. Gaby, *Preventing and Reversing Osteoporosis* (Rocklin, Calif.: Prima Publishing, 1994), 166, 167; and Ray Sahelian, *DHEA, A Practical Guide* (Garden City Park, N.Y.: Avery Publishing Group, 1996), 59–64.

2. Regelson and Colman, *The Super-Hormone Promise*, 20.

3. M. M. Iwu et al., "Hypoglycaemic Activity of Dioscoretine from Tubers of *Dioscorea dumetorum* in Normal and Alloxan Diabetic Rabbits, *Plante Medica* 56 (1990): 264–67, quoted in Stephen Nugent, "Plants That Make Hormones (Part II)," *The Nugent Report* 4, no. 6 (June 1997): 4.

4. *Magic and Medicine of Plants* (New York: Reader's Digest, 1993), 341.

5. John R. Lee, *What Your Doctor May* Not *Tell You About Menopause* (New York: Warner Books, 1996), 300.

6. Ibid., 300, 301.

7. Julian Whitaker, "Clear Up Inflammation with Enzymes," *Dr. Julian Whitaker's Health and Healing*, 8, no. 8 (August 1998): 1. See also Trien Susan Falmholtz, *Change of Life* (New York: Fawcett Columbine Books, 1986); James F. Balch and Phyllis A. Balch, *Prescription for Nutritional Healing* (Garden City Park, N.Y.: Avery Publishing Group, 1990), 142.

8. Skye Lininger et al., *The Natural Pharmacy* (Rocklin, Calif.: Prima Health, 1998), 320.

9. Iwu et al., "Hypoglycaemic Activity of Dioscoretine from Tubers of *Dioscorea dumetorum* in Normal and Alloxan Diabetic Rabbits," 264–67, quoted in Nugent, "Plants that Make Hormones (Part II)," 1.

10. For information on diosgenin's ability to decrease cholesterol in the liver, see M. R. Malinow, *New York Academy of Science* 454, (1985): 23; M. N. Cayen et al., *Journal of Lipid Research* 20 (1979): 174; K. Uchida et al., *Journal of Lipid Research* 25 (1984): 236; M. R. Malinow et al., *Journal of Lipid Research* 28 (1987): 1; J. Laguna et al., *Journal of Atherosclerosis* 2 (1962): 459; and Yves Sauvaire et al., "Implication of Steroid Saponins and Sapogenins in the Hypocholesterolemic Effect of Fenugreek," *Lipids* 26, no. 3 (1991): 191–97. For information on diosgenin's ability to lower blood pressure, see H. Tsukatari et al., *Journal of Neurochemistry* 44 (1985): 658. For information on the ability of diosgenin to aid in adrenal function, see Philip Stavish, "DHEA: The Rejuvenating Hormone," 3, no. 8 (1997): 43.

11. H. D. Kikino et al., *Planta Medica* (1986): 168.

12. Stephen Nugent, "Plants that Make Hormones (Part II)." *The Nugent Report* 4, no. 6, June 1997, 3.

13. Iwu et al., "Hypoglycaemic Activity of Dioscoretine from Tubers of *Dioscorea Dumetorum* in Normal and Alloxan Diabetic Rabbits," 264–67, cited in Nugent, "Plants that Make Hormones (Part 11)," 3.

14. Michael Warshaw and M. W. Lab, "Natural Progesterone," *World Health News*, Fall 1997, 38.

15. Nugent, "Plants that Make Hormones," 3; and A. Rao, A. R. Rao, and R. K. Kale, "Diosgenin—A Growth Stimulator of Mammary Gland of Ovariectomized Mouse," *Indian Journal of Experimental Biology* 30 (1992): 367.

16. For information on *Dioscorea villosa*'s ability to increase bone density, see G. Kaata et al., "Emprise Optimal Health Plan," *Emprise Adventurer Magazine* 1 (1996): 14–15. For information on how *Dioscorea villosa* works as an antioxidant, see M. Araghiniknam et al., "Antioxidant Activity of Dioscorea and Dehydroepiandrosterone (DHEA) in Older Humans," *Life Sciences* 11 (1996): 147–57.

17. Rao, Rao, and Kale, "Diosgenin—A Growth Stimulator," 367.

18. Nugent, "Plants that Make Hormones," 4. See also J. L. Bencytout et al., "A Plant Steroid, Diosgenin, a New Megakaryocytic Differentiation Inducer of Hel Cells," *Biochemical Biophysical Research Communication* 207, no. 1 (1995): 398–404.

19. Philip Stavish, "DHEA: The Rejuvenating Hormone," 43.

20. Nugent, "Plants that Make Hormones," 3.

21. Regelson and Colman, *The Super-Hormone Promise*, 34.

22. Steve Sternberg, "Tracking Biological Sabotage," *USA Today*, 16 September 1997, Science section, p. 4D.

23. B. A. Araneo et al., "Reversal of the Immunosenecent Phenotype by Dehydroepiandrosterone: Hormone Treatment Provides an Adjuvant Effect on the Immunization of Aged Mice with Recombinant Hepatitis B Surface Antigen," *Journal of Infectious Diseases* 167 (1993): 830–40.

24. Betty Kamen, "Fibromyalgia: An Age-Old Malady Begging for Respect," *Let's Live*, November 1994, 31.

25. Richard P. Huemer, "Fibromyalgia: The Pain That Never Stops," *Let's Live*, November 1996, 34–35.

26. Balch and Balch, *Prescription for Nutritional Healing*, 274.

27. Raquel Martin and Judi Gerstung, *The Estrogen Alternative: Natural Hormone Therapy with Botanical Progesterone*, 3rd ed. (Rochester, Vt.: Healing Arts Press, 1997), 66–68.

28. Peat, *From PMS to Menopause*, 2.

29. S. S. Jick et al., "Risk of Idiopathic Cerebral Haemorrhage in Women on Oral Contraceptives with Differing Progestagen Components," *Lancet* 354 (1999): 302–3.

30. John R. Lee, *What Your Doctor May* Not *Tell You About Menopause* (New York: Warner Books, 1996), 64.

31. R. Peat and A. L. Soderwall, "Cold-Inactivated Enzymes," *Physiological Chemistry and Physics* (1972).

32. Peat, *From PMS to Menopause*, 64.

33. Ibid., 112.

34. Lee, *Natural Progesterone*, 6, 35.

35. Peat, *From PMS to Menopause*, 63.

36. John R. Lee, "Significance of Molecular Configuration Specificity— The Case of Progesterone and Osteoporosis," *Townsend Letter for Doctors* (June 1993): 558.

37. For information on progesterone and bone formation, see J. C. Prior, "Progesterone as a Bone-Trophic Hormone," *Endocrine Reviews* 11, no. 2 (1990): 386–98. For information on progesterone and the reduction of bone loss, see E. L. Berengolts et al., "Effects of Progesterone on Post-Ovariectomy Bone Loss in Aged Rats," *Journal of Bone and Mineral Research* 5 (1990): 1143–47; and J. C. Prior et al., "Spinal Bone Loss and Ovulatory Disturbances," *International Journal of Gynaecology and Obstetries* 34 (1990): 253–56. For information on progesterone and a decreased risk of osteoporosis, see Lee, *What Your Doctor May* Not *Tell You*, 159–68; and Gaby, *Preventing and Reversing Osteoporosis*, 143–46.

38. Edward McDonagh, "Can Chiropractic Reverse Osteoporosis," *The Internist* 2, no. IV (December 1995): 19, 20.

39. Ibid.

40. Peat, *From PMS to Menopause*, 110.

41. Lee, *What Your Doctor May* Not *Tell You*, 40–42, 71, 72, 80; and Martin and Gerstung, *The Estrogen Alternative*, 24–26, 45–46.

42. Martin and Gerstung, *The Estrogen Alternative*, 76–77.

43. Lita Lee, "Estrogen, Progesterone and Female Problems," *Earthletter*, 1, no. 2 (June 1991).

44. Peat, *From PMS to Menopause*, 113.

45. Peat, *From PMS to Menopause*, 113, quote on 114.

46. Ibid., 114.

47. Lee, *What Your Doctor May* Not *Tell You*, 8, 52.

48. Anne Dickson and Nikki Henriques, *Women on Menopause* (Rochester, Vt.: Healing Arts Press, 1988), 94.

49. Lee, *What Your Doctor May* Not *Tell You*, 158.

50. Regelson and Colman, *The Super-Hormone Promise*, 41.

51. Peter Casson, *Youth Hormone* (Medical Breakthroughs Ivanhoe Broadcast News, 1997), broadcast news interview transcript with Q&A #853, www.ivanhoe.com/backissues/youthhormone.html.

52. Dallas Clouatre, *Anti-Fat Nutrients* (San Francisco: Pax Publishing, 1995), 45.

53. Gaby, *Preventing and Reversing Osteoporosis*, 164.

54. Ibid., 167.

55. Andrew A. Skolnick, "Scientific Verdict Still Out on DHEA," *Medical News & Perspectives* (6 November 1996): 5 (www.ama-assn.org/sci-pubs/journals/archive/jama/vol_276/no_17/mn6188.htm).

56. Regelson and Colman, *The Super-Hormone Promise*, 84.

57. Julian Whitaker, "DHEA Helps to Regulate the Immune System," *Dr. Julian Whitaker's Health and Healing*, 8, no. 9 (September 1998): 5. See also R. F. van Vollenhoven et al., "Treatment of Systemic Lupus Erythematosus with Dehydroepiandrosterone: 50 Patients Treated up to 12 Months," *Journal of Rheumatology* 25 (1998): 285–89; and B. C. Tilley et al., "Minocycline in Rheumatoid Arthritis. A 48-Week, Double-Blind, Placebo-Controlled Trial," *Annals of Internal Medicine* 122, no. 2 (1995): 81–89.

58. Whitaker, "DHEA Helps to Regulate the Immune System," 5. See also T. Suzuki et al., "Low Serum Levels of Dehydroepiandrosterone May Cause Deficient IL-2 Production by Lymphocytes in Patients with Systemic Lupus Erythematosus (SLE)," *Clinical Experimental Immunology* 99 (1995): 251–55.

59. Richard P. Huemer, M.D. "Fibromyalgia: The Pain That Never Stops," 35.

60. "Genelabs Says DHEA Benefits Lupus Patients," *Reuters*, 1996.

61. R. F. van Vollenhoven et al., "An Open Study of Dehydroepiandros-terone in Systemic Lupus Erythematosus," *Arthritis and Rheumatism* 37, no. 9 (1994): 1305–10.

62. Regelson and Colman, *The Super-Hormone Promise*.

63. Casson, *Youth Hormone*, Q&A #908.

64. Joe Glickman, Jr., "Hormone Holds Key to Aging Process," *Health Science Report* 2, no. 1 (1996): 2.

65. J. F. Mortola, *Journal of Clinical Endocrinology* 71, no. 3, 696–704.

66. For information on DHEA and organ health, see Arlene J. Morales et al., "Effects of Replacement Dose of Dehydroepiandrosterone in Men

and Women of Advancing Age," *Journal of Clinical Endocrinology and Metabolism* 78, no. 6 (1994): 1360–67. For information on DHEA and atherosclerosis, heart disease, and strokes, see *Journal of Clinical Endocrinology* 66 no. 1 (1988): 57–61; and *Journal of Clinical Investigation* 82, no. 2 (1988): 712–20. For information on DHEA and the immune system, see Barbara Araneo and Raymond Daynes, "Dehydroepiandrosterone Functions As More than an Antiglucocorticoid in Preserving Immunocompetence after Thermal Injury," *Endocrinology* 136, no. 2 (1995): 393–401.

67. Dean Raffelock, "Why Good Liver Function Makes for Better Hormone Balance," *The John R. Lee, M.D., Medical Letter,* (September 1999): 5.

68. D. Ben-Nathan, *Archives of Virology* 120, no. 3–4 (1991): 263–71; and E. Henderson et al., "Dehydroepiandrosterone and 16-alpha-bromoepiandrosterone: Inhibitors of Epstein-Barr Virus-induced Transformation of Human Lymphocytes," *Carcinogenesis* 2, no. 7 (1981): 683–86.

69. Hanna Kroeger, *God Helps Those Who Help Themselves* (Boulder, Colo.: Hanna Kroeger Publications, 1996), 219.

70. A. G. Schwartz, *Cancer Research* 48, no. 17 (1988): 4817–22; Casson, *Youth Hormone*, Q&A #853; and Skolnick, "Scientific Verdict Still Out on DHEA."

71. Clouatre, *Anti-Fat Nutrients*, 45. See also A. A. Tagliaferro et al., "The Effect of Dehydroepiandrosterone (DHEA) on Calorie Intake, Body Weight, and Resting Metabolism," *Federation Proceeding* (abstract 201) 42 (1983): 326; and K. Yoshimoto et al., "Reciprocal Effects of Epidermal Growth Factor on Key Lipogenic Enzymes in Primary Cultures of Adult Rat Hepatocytes. Induction of Glucose-6-Phosphate Dehydrogenase and Suppression of Malic Enzyme and Lipogenesis," *Journal of Biological Chemisty* 258 (1983): 1255.

72. Clouatre, *Anti-Fat Nutrients*, 45. See also Julian Whitaker, "New Hope on Obesity and Diabetes," *Dr. Julian Whitaker's Health and Healing* 2, no. 11 (October 1992): 4–5; D. L. Coleman et al., "Effect of Genetic Background on the Therapeutic Effects of DHEA in Diabetes-Obesity Mutants in Aged Normal Mice," *Diabetes* 33 (1984): 26; and Douglas L. Coleman, "Antiobesity Effects of Etiocholanolones in Diabetes (Db), Viable Yellow and Normal Mice," *Endocrinology* 117, no. 6 (1985): 2279–83.

73. Alan E. Lewis, "Melatonin: Part 2," *Consumer Bulletin, Whole Foods*, March 1996, 102; and D. E. Blask et al., "Melatonin Action on Oncogenesis," in *Role of Melatonin and Pineal Peptides in*

*Neuroimmunomodulation*, ed. F. Fraschini and R. J. Reiter (New York: Plenum, 1991), 233–40.

74.  Gaby, *Preventing and Reversing Osteoporosis*, 61.

75.  Eugene Roberts, "The 'Charm' of Pregnenolone," interview by the Editor, *Life Enhancement News* issue 24 (August 1996): 20; and Ray Sahelian, *Pregnenolone*, (Marina Del Rey, Calif.: Melatonin/DHEA Research Institute, 1996), 3.

76.  Paavo O. Airola, *There Is a Cure for Arthritis* (West Nyack, N.Y.: Parker Publishing Company, 1968), 37.

77.  Raymond Peat, *Nutrition for Women* (Eugene, Oreg.: International University, 1981).

78.  Lee, *What Your Doctor May Not Tell You*, 258.

79.  Peat, *From PMS to Menopause*, 13.

80.  Ibid., 61, 114; G. G. Bole et al., "Rheumatic Symptoms and Serological Abnormalities Induced by Oral Contraceptive," *Lancet* 1 (1969): 323; C. Christiansen, "The Different Routes of Administration and the Effect of Hormone Replacement Therapy on Osteoporosis," *Fertility and Sterility* 62, no. 6 (supplement 2) (1994): S152–S156; and "Consider, if Hyperprolactinemia Leads to Osteopenia, and the Administration of Estrogens to Postmenopausal Women Leads to Hyperprolactinemia," *Yearbook of Endocrinology* (1984): 273.

81.  Peat, *From PMS to Menopause*, 15.

82.  C. Rodriquez et al., "Estrogen Replacement Therapy and Fatal Ovarian Cancer," *American Journal of Epidemiology* 141 (1995): 828–34. See also L. A. Brinton et al., "Oral Contraceptives and Breast Cancer Risk Among Younger Women," *Journal of the National Cancer Institute* 98, no. 11 (1995): 827–35; E. L. Cavalieri et al., "Molecular Origin of Cancer; Catechol Estrogen-3, 4-quinones as Endogenous Tumor Initiators," *Proceedings of the National Academy of Sciences* 94 (1994): 10937–42; Robert F. Service, "New Role for Estrogen in Cancer?" *Science* 179 (1998): 1631–33; and J. Fischman et al., "The Role of Estrogen in Mammary Carcinogenesis," *Annals of the New York Academy of Sciences* 768, no. 91 (1995).

83.  T. Ushiyama et al., "Expression of Estrogen Receptor Related Protein (p29) and Estradiol Binding in Human Arthritic Synovium," *Journal of Rheumatology* 22 (1995): 421–26; and T. D. Koepsell et al., "Non-Contraceptive Hormones and the Risk of Rheumatoid Arthritis in Menopausal Women," *International Journal of Epidemiology* 23, no. 6 (1994): 1248–55.

84. Raymond Peat, *Ray Peat's Newsletter,* 1995. See also Ushiyama et al., "Expression of Estrogen Receptor Related Protein," 421–26.

85. Jorge Sanchez-Guerrero et al., "Past Use of Oral Contraceptives and the Risk of Developing Systemic Lupus Erythematosus," *Arthritis and Rheumatism* 40, no. 5 (May 1997): 804–08, cited in John R. Lee, "Even the Low Dose Pill Is Dangerous," *The John R. Lee, M.D. Medical Letter* (November 1998): 4.

86. Peat, *Ray Peat's Newsletter,* 1995; Peat, *From PMS to Menopause,* 45. See also B. V. Stadel, "Oral Contraceptives and Cardiovascular Disease," *New England Journal of Medicine* 305 (1981): 612; M. P. Vessey et al., "Investigation of Relation Between Use of Oral Contraceptives and Thromboembolic Disease," *British Medical Journal* 2 (1968): 199–205; P. W. F. Wilson et al., "Postmenopausal Estrogen Use, Cigarette Smoking, and Cardiovascular Morbidity in Women over 50," *New England Journal of Medicine* 313, no. 17 (1985): 1038–43; L. A. Noris et al., "Effect of Oestrogen Dose on Whole Blood Platelet Activation in Women Taking New Low Dose Oral Contraceptives," *Thrombosis and Haemostasis* 72, no. 6 (1994): 926–30; S. M. Goodrich et al., "Effect of Estradiol 17b on Peripheral Venous Blood Flow," *American Journal of Obstetrics and Gynecology* 96 (1966): 407; B. B. Gerstman et al., "Oral Contraceptive Estrogen Dose and the Risk of Deep Venous Thromboembolic Disease," *American Journal of Epidemiology* 133 (1991): 32–36; and M. Thorogood, "The Epidemiology of Cardiovascular Disease in Relation to the Estrogen Dose of Oral Contraceptives: A Historical Perspective," *Advances in Contraception* 7 (supplement 3) (1991): 11–21.

87. G. Holdstock et. al., "Effects of Testosterone, Oestradiol and Progesterone on Immune Regulation," *Clinical and Experimental Immunology* 47 (1982): 449–56.

88. Lee, *What Your Doctor May Not Tell You,* 26, 86, 89, 119–23, 162–63.

89. Prior et al., "Spinal Bone Loss and Ovulatory Disturbances," 253–56. See also Prior, "Progesterone as a Bone-Trophic Hormone," 386–98; and John R. Lee, "Significance of Molecular Configuration Specificity—The Case of Progesterone and Osteoporosis," *Townsend Letter for Doctors* (June 1993): 558.

90. John R. Lee, "David Zava's New Lab and New Formula for Assessing Hormone Balance," *The John R. Lee, M.D. Medical Letter* (November 1998).

91. Lee, *What Your Doctor May Not Tell You;* and Betty Kamen, *Hormone Replacement Therapy: YES or NO?* (Novato, Calif.: Nutrition Encounter, 1993).

92. For information on immunological balance, see "Autoimmunity: The Female Connection," *Medscape Women's Health* 1, no. 11 (1996). (www.medscapte.com/Clinical/Medscape/womens.health/1996/vol.nll/w207.merrill/ref-w207.merrill.html).

93. Schumacher M. Koenig et al., "Progesterone Synthesis and Myelin Formation by Schwann Cells: A Newly Demonstrated Role of Progesterone," *Science* 268, no. 5216 (1995): 1500–03.

94. Roberts, "The 'Charm' of Pregnenolone," 16.

95. Billie J. Sahley, "Pregnenolone," *Health Store News*, April/May 1997, 9.

96. Koenig et al., "Progesterone Synthesis and Myelin Formation," 1500–1503.

97. Ibid.

98. Lee, *What Your Doctor May Not Tell You*, 95.

99. Regelson and Colman, *The Super-Hormone Promise*, 188.

100. Lee, *What Your Doctor May Not Tell You*, 61. "American Home Video Natural Medicine Update," (1995 TV program on the subject of hormone replacement therapy with guest Betty Kamen, Ph.D., hosts Jeffrey and Valerie Donigan.)

101. "Natural Medicine Update."

102. Ibid.

103. Lloyd Guth et al., "Key Role for Pregnenolone in Combination Therapy that Promotes Recovery After Spinal Cord Injury," *Proceedings of the National Academy of Sciences* 91 (1994): 12308–12; and Koenig, "Progesterone Synthesis and Myelin Formation," 1500–03.

104. Regelson and Colman, *The Super-Hormone Promise*, 111.

105. Lloyd Guth et al., "Key Role for Pregnenolone," 12308–12; and Koenig et al., "Progesterone Synthesis and Myelin Formation," 1500–03.

106. Roberts, "The 'Charm' of Pregnenolone," 19.

107. Regelson and Colman, *The Super-Hormone Promise*, 110.

108. E. Henderson et al., "Pregnenolone," *Journal of Clinical Endocrinology* 10 (1950): 455–74, cited in Sahelian, *Pregnenolone*, (Garden City Park, N.Y.: Avery Publishing Group, 1997), 59.

109. "News Update," *Women's Health Advocate Newsletter* 4, no. 11 (January 1998): 1.

110. Roberts, "The 'Charm' of Pregnenolone," 15, 16.

111. Koenig, et al., "Progesterone Synthesis and Myelin Formation by Schwann Cells," 1500–03, cited in Sahelian, *Pregnenolone*, 67.

112. E. Henderson, et al., "Pregnenolone," 455–74, cited in Sahelian, *Pregnenolone*, 67.

113. Ibid, 60.

114. H. Freeman et al., "Therapeutic Efficacy of Delta-5 Pregnenolone in Rheumatoid Arthritis," *Journal of the American Medical Association* (1950): 1124–28, quote on 1124.

115. Ibid., 1124–28.

116. Henderson, Weinberg, and Wright, "Pregnenolone," 455–74; and Sahelian, *Pregnenolone* (Garden City Park, N.Y.: Avery Publishing Group, 1997), 19.

117. Sahelian, *Pregnenolone*, 86–89.

118. Ibid., 125–30.

119. Ibid., 59.

120. Regelson and Colman, *The Super-Hormone Promise*, 111.

121. Roberts, "The 'Charm' of Pregnenolone," 20.

122. Sahelian, *Pregnenolone* (Garden City Park, N.Y.: Avery Publishing Group, 1997), 97, 98.

123. Editorial, *Journal of American Medical Association* (September 1966), cited in Paavo O. Airola, *There Is a Cure for Arthritis* (West Nyack, N.Y.: Parker Publishing Company, 1968), 39.

124. Floyd S. Daft, *U.S. News and World Report* (June 3, 1955), cited in Airola, *There Is a Cure for Arthritis*, 39.

125. Regelson and Colman, *The Super-Hormone Promise*, 111, cited in Airola, *There Is a Cure for Arthritis*, 39.

126. R. P. Watterson, "Arthritis, Biochemical Suffocation," *Southwestern Medicine* 42, no. 4 (April 1961), cited in Airola, *There Is a Cure for Arthritis*, 39.

127. Julian Whitaker, "A Natural Substance That May Prevent Paralysis: Pregnenolone Has Likely Been Around as Long as You Have," *Dr. Julian Whitaker's Health and Healing* 5, no. 2 (February 1995): 2.

128. Sahelian, *Pregnenolone* (Marina Del Rey, Calif.: Melatonin/DHEA Research Institute, 1996), 3.

129. Ibid., 13.

130. Regelson and Colman, *The Super-Hormone Promise*, 103, 104.

131. Guth et al., "Key Role for Pregnenolone," 12308–12, quote on 12311.

132. Hans Selye et al., "Potentiation of a Pituitary Extract with Pregnenolone and Additional Observations Concerning the Influence of Various Organs on Steroid Metabolism, *Rev Can Biol* 2 (1943): 319–328, cited in Sahelian, *Pregnenolone* (Marina Del Rey, Calif.: Melatonin/DHEA Research Institute, 1996), 5.

133. Eugene Roberts, "The 'Charm' of Pregnenolone," 21.

134. Regelson and Colman, *The Super-Hormone Promise*, 204.

135. Ibid., 104.

136. Ibid., 155.

137. Skolnick, "Scientific Verdict Still Out on DHEA."

138. Raffelock, "Why Good Liver Function," 6.

139. R. Davison et al., "Effects of delta 5 Pregnenolone in Rheumatoid Arthritis," *Archives of Internal Medicine* 85 (1950): 365–88; and Freeman et al., "Therapeutic Efficacy of Delta-5 Pregnenolone," 1124.

140. Martin and Gerstung, *The Estrogen Alternative*.

141. Regelson and Colman, *The Super-Hormone Promise*, 110.

142. Katharina Dalton, *Once a Month* (Pomona, Calif.: Hunter House, 1979), 182. See also Regelson and Colman, *The Super-Hormone Promise*, 103, 108.

143. Peat, *From PMS to Menopause*, 74.

144. Lee et al., *What Your Doctor May Not Tell You About Menopause*, 322.

145. Lee, *Natural Progesterone*, 78, 264–265, 267.

146. Dalton, *Once a Month*, 145.

147. Peat, *From PMS to Menopause*, 74.

## Chapter 7

1. Peter H. Gott, "Is Your Doctor Over-Doctoring You?" *Redbook*, October 1987, 112.

2. L. Galland, *Basic Concepts, Diagnostics and Therapeutic Techniques in Functional Medicine* (Gig Harbor, Wash.: HealthComm, 1996).

3. The Burton Goldberg Group, *Alternative Medicine* (Puyallup, Wash.: Future Medicine Publishing, 1993), 27. 159–877.

4. Stuart M. Berger, *What Your Doctor Didn't Learn in Medical School* (New York: William Morrow, 1988): 13.

5. Alicia Evans, "Natural Remedies Are Superior," *Atlanta Journal and Constitution*, 26 March 1999, A19.

6. For more information on nutraceuticals, contact the American Nutraceutical Association, 22 Inverness Center Parkway, Suite 150, Birmingham, AL 35242; (205) 980-5710; www. americanutra.com.

7. Berger, *What Your Doctor Didn't Learn in Medical School*, 13.

8. Ibid., 13, 236; and Burton Goldberg Group, *Alternative Medicine*, 17.

9. Burton Goldberg Group, *Alternative Medicine*, 17.

10. Peter J. D'Adamo, *Eat Right for Your Type* (New York: G. P. Putnam's Sons, 1996) 97.

11. *FACTS Bulletin*, vol. 3 (Foundation for the Advancement of Chiropractic Tenets and Science, 1990).

12. Sid E. Williams, *Chiropractic in the American Health-Care System* (Marietta, Ga.: Life Chiropractic College,1986).

13. George P. McAndrews et al., *Finally after 11 Years the Federal Court in Chicago, Illinois Found the American Medical Association GUILTY!!!* (Huntington Beach, Calif.: Motion Palpation Institute, 1987), 8.

14. Ibid.

15. George P. McAndrews, "Guilty: United States Court of Apeals Upholds Judge Getzendanner's Judgment in Wilk Anti-trust Suit," *MPI's Dynamic Chiropractic*, 48, no. 5 (1990): 14.

16. McAndrews, et al., *Finally After 11 Years*, 22, 23.

17. Raquel Martin, *Today's Health Alternative* (Tehachapi, Calif.: America West Publishers, 1992), 106–107.

18. James J. Locker, Letter to the editor, *Atlanta Journal and Constitution*, 6 September, 1987.

19. Elliott Segal, "Chiropractic Lay Lecture," audiotape.

20. Victor Hugo, *Story of a Crime*, cited in Joseph E. Maynard, *Healing Hands* (Woodstock, Ga.: Jonorm Publishing Company, 1991).

21. Thomas J. Moore, *Prescription for Disaster* (New York: Simon & Schuster, 1998), 15.

## Epilogue

1. Jeffrey S. Bland, *The Inflammatory Disorders* (Gig Harbor, Wash.: HealthComm, 1997) 27.

2. Rachelle Vinet Sellner, "Monsieur Vinet," (family biography, Huntingdon Valley, Pa. 1973), 183. My grandfather, Professeur Camille Vinet, came to this country from France to teach Latin, algebra, geometry, physics, and of course French. His true aim was to contemplate the infinite power we have at our command.

3. Emanuel Swedenborg, *Heaven and Its Wonders and Hell* (London: Swedenborg Society, 1937), 54–62.

# Index